AYURVEDA'S THREE PILLARS OF HEALTH

A MAP TO HEALTH, RESILIENCE, AND WELL-BEING

MONA L. WARNER

Publishing services provided by 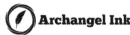 **Archangel Ink**

ISBN-13: 978-1-9994272-3-8

Gummo—This is your book. I really hope you like it.
Thank you.

Chère grand-maman—I miss you. You were my favourite
walking talking book, *notre encyclopedie ambulatrice.*

To Grannie—The books you gifted me every year were the
greatest gift. Thank you for the inspiration to write my own.

Contents

Note from the Author

Dear Reader,

Welcome to this journey through the basic principles of a healing science I hold very near and dear to my heart, Ayurveda (pronounced "ah-yur-vey-duh").

I came to Ayurveda not from a place of intellectual curiosity (at least not at first) but from a place of depletion, depression, and desperation. Sounds bad and yet, thanks to Ayurveda, it's all good.

I was never a particularly robust human being. My mom says that when I was born, my skin reacted strongly to the air, and I was beet red for weeks. From there, I was a colicky baby (sorry, Mom). By the time I was four years old, the doctors told my mom I was anaemic, and so began our regimen of eating liver three times a week. At the age of six, I was pre-scribed glasses and not just for reading. All through school, I caught every cold and flu that was going around. In my teens, I did okay. Then college happened, and by the time I was 23 years old, I started having seizures. By 26, I had to leave my job because I was so out of sorts that I could not keep working; it was too much.

My doctors and specialists did the best they could with the tools they had, and I am grateful for their wisdom, sugges-tions, and support. As it turned out, though, those approaches didn't work for me.

It took years before I stumbled upon Ayurveda, and then it was quite by accident! Ayurveda is an ancient medical science that originated in India over five thousand years ago and is still in practice today. The Sanskrit word *Ayurveda* translates to "living wisdom." *Ayus* or *Ayur* translate to "life," and *veda* translates to "knowledge" or "wisdom." It is a set of teachings, tools, and practices that maintain the health of the healthy[1] and restore the health of the sick when it can. That said, regardless of which medical system you are working with, some diseases are incurable. Ayurveda promotes health through practices that cultivate balance, stability, and peace in the body, mind, and spirit; as such, it is a science of longevity.

With ten years of Ayurveda under my belt, things are very different for me today. I own a yoga school and teach weekly yoga classes. I offer yoga teacher trainings, teaching others how to teach yoga. I teach Ayurveda in workshops, at conferences, and in other yogis' trainings and programs. I studied formally for six years to become a Certified Ayurvedic Practitioner, which allows me to work one-on-one with people to help them find health and balance in their own lives so they can thrive ... and that's just my work life. My husband and I love to travel and explore. We have a dog who is active, a cat who is cat-like, and families and friends. My life is rich, full, and beautiful. Thanks to Ayurveda I can embrace and enjoy it, standing in my own health. The teachings of Ayurveda (plus yoga) enable me to be strong and resilient, feeling good in my body-mind. Ayurveda helped me heal many of my health challenges, and it helps me support others to do the same. This

---

1   From the *Charaka Samhita, Sutrasthana 30.26.*

allows me to live my life. I have to pay attention and listen, and now I know what to listen for and how to respond.

Why Did I Pick Ayurveda?

That's a great question. There are many health and healing modalities to pursue, so why did I choose this one? Truth is, I fell into it. It started showing up for me in 2008. An Ayurvedic doctor came to town for a visit. He offered a course in *marma* therapy, which I took. Then it was part of a yoga teacher training that I signed up for, and this is where the magic happened. I was introduced to the Ayurvedic daily routine. Like a good student, I did it. In the course of one week, I started to notice significant differences in my body and mind … and I knew I was onto something. So I kept practicing a little every day. I got stronger and healthier, a little every day. Sure, there were ups and downs—it's life—there's no escaping this. Yet with each daily routine practice, I got healthier, stronger, and more resilient.

I really appreciate that Ayurveda has been practiced for thousands of years. I figure if it didn't work, people would have stopped using it. There is a deep, time-tested wisdom in these teachings, and for me, these practices really make a difference in my body and mind. The teachings are profound, and there came a point where I needed a guide to help me along my path. I signed up to take the Foundations of Ayurveda program at the Kripalu School of Ayurveda.

When I began my formal study of Ayurveda, I was deeply inspired by its definition of health, which you'll find below. Prior to this, I had unconsciously defined health as the absence of disease, and yet that wasn't quite right. Just because I wasn't having a seizure didn't mean I felt good in my body or focused in my mind.

Inspiration

The inspiration for this book, and my passion for teaching Ayurveda, are rooted in the Ayurvedic definition of *health*. I learned a passage from the Ayurvedic classical texts and not only did I love the Sanskrit chant, I was so grateful for its meaning and guidance.

I don't plan to use a ton of Sanskrit in this book; however, there will be keywords included and translated. *Shloka* is the Sanskrit word that refers to a passage or teaching from one of the classical texts. The classical texts are the books that house the Ayurvedic teachings. The classical texts are listed in the **Further Reading** section at the end for those who are interested.

The passage that completely changed how I looked at the concept of health is known as the *svastha shloka*, which translates to *passage on the definition of health*. First, the Sanskrit:

Sama dosha sama agnischa sama dhatu mala kriyaḥ
Prasanna atma indriya manaḥ svastha iti abhidhiyate[2]

The translation of this passage from the classical text known as the *Sushruta Samhita* is:

Balanced constitution *(sama dosha)*, balanced digestive

---

2   From the *Sushruta Samhita, Sutrasthana 15.41.*

4

fire *(sama agnischa)*, balanced tissues *(sama dhatu)*, and the proper elimination of wastes *(mala kriyaḥ)*

Blissfulness *(prasanna)* in the soul *(atma)*, senses *(indriya)*, and mind *(manaḥ)*,

This is what we call *(iti abhidhiyate)* health *(svastha)*

This Ayurvedic definition of health is comprehensive and multidimensional. It is about more than the absence of disease. It is also, in a way, a moving target. There are many factors involved in creating a context or situation in our lives that promotes health.

This book is about Ayurveda's three pillars of health:[3]

1. Nourishment

2. Sleep

3. Energy Management

These pillars were established to balance all the elements of our physical body (constitution, digestive potential, tissues, and wastes) in order to create a sense of blissfulness in the soul, the senses, and in the mind.

All of this comes together to create what we call *health*.

Based on the passage above, we now know that the Sanskrit word *svastha* translates to health. I want to take a moment to break down the word *svastha* itself, which will expand upon our idea of health.

---

3   From the *Ashtanga Samgraha, Sutrasthana 9.18* and the *Charaka Samhita, Sutrasthana 11.35*.

The first part of the word, *sva*, translates to "self." The second part of the word, *stha*, translates to "stability." The translation of the complete word *svastha* is "seated in the self" or "stable in one's self." So even if you can't remember all the parts of the longer translation, health is found when we are established in our self.

By being seated in the center of our own self, we are able to connect to the wisdom and knowing that exists within us. Some will refer to this as their inner teacher, spirit, guide, guru, or intuition. Call it whatever you want. ☺ The idea is to connect to this inner wisdom and make choices from this place. It leads us to maintain the health we have and to continue optimizing and moving toward an even healthier state of being.

The primary goal of Ayurveda is to *maintain the health of the healthy person*. In a lecture I listened to, Dr. Robert Svoboda said, "There is really no limit to the degree of balance that a sincere harmony-seeker can achieve from the practice of Ayurveda." How awesome is that? We can use these tools to get healthy, and we can use these tools to stay healthy. It is, in my experience, easier to maintain your health than it is to build it. Either way, working toward a state of health is a very worthwhile investment.

My Intention

I created this book to share the basic concepts of Ayurveda with my clients, and others who aren't familiar with Ayurveda, using the map of the three pillars of health. This is a great starting point for anyone who wants to see if the Ayurvedic approach makes sense and works for them.

In my Ayurvedic practice I often hear that people want to work with Ayurveda, but they get stuck because they cannot figure out their constitution, known in Sanskrit as *dosha*. I want to offer a resource that invites you to try Ayurveda even if you don't know, can't figure out, or don't care about your *dosha*.

I wanted to write a practical everyday Ayurveda guide that wasn't centered on the *doshas*. Given Ayurveda's definition of health and that balancing *dosha* is the first step to health, I recognize that *dosha* is an important (and amazing) concept in Ayurveda. What I also realize is that it can take years to understand *doshas* thoroughly. I found most people knew enough about *doshas* to get into trouble and not enough to get back out. Then they would claim that Ayurveda did not work when, really, their incomplete understanding did not work.

With this in mind, I started to look at my Ayurveda practice differently, with more curiosity and openness, and I noticed something. I noticed there were a lot of things that could be done to support people regardless of what their *dosha* was or whether they had figured out their *doshas*. When I paid even closer attention, I realized these threads of practice common to everyone were beautifully woven into a different Ayurvedic map—not the *dosha* map but the three pillars of health map.

And thus was born the idea for this book, an Ayurveda book that supports you through the three pillars of health, whether you know your *dosha* or not. Ironically, using these ideas and strengthening and supporting the three pillars of health will bring balance—*then* your *dosha* will reveal itself. 😌 Isn't that ironic? You gotta love the universe.

Once you give it a try, if Ayurveda makes sense to you, I highly recommend finding an Ayurvedic Health Counsellor, Ayurvedic Practitioner, or doctor in your area to work with. Along with the definition of health, Ayurveda school taught me that the Ayurvedic teachings are profound, useful, and health promoting. It also taught me that we are best served having a guide on our journey through the teachings. There is much depth to these teachings, and it gets easy to zoom in on one thing, forgetting all the other pieces of the puzzle. Although the recommendations I give in this book will get you started, you'll benefit greatly from working one-on-one with someone who can help fine-tune the program and process. Also, we can't see what we can't see about ourselves. We all have blind spots, so having a set of outside eyes is really useful in terms of making progress along our path.

How to Use This Book

My suggestion is to read this book in order. I have laid it out so that the information builds as we go. The first section starts with the basic concepts of Ayurveda, things you need to know in order to understand the three pillars of health. Then I talk through each pillar in detail: how they work and what is included in each pillar. Notice how the passage about the definition of health is interwoven through the pillars, and how these fit together in a beautiful and poetic way. 💜

Each section of the book is filled with recommendations you can use to choose health every day. I'm talking about simple daily choices like tongue scraping, chewing your food, and going to bed on time. Remember that each pillar leans on the previous one, so the book is written in sequence. My hope is that the format of the book not only gives you options but also understanding around why these things are important. The why allows you to choose the things that you need to bring more balance and health into your life.

As you read the book, you might notice that some recommendations are useful to support many different aspects of your health—by this I mean that one recommendation might be offered multiple times and in more than one section of the book. This is going to create some noticeable repetition. I chose the repetition for a few reasons:

1. Repetition helps us remember. If a recommendation does a ton of great stuff for you, I want you to remember it!

2. I want you to notice which recommendations are useful for multiple things.

3. I wanted you to find the recommendations in the sections they are pertinent to without having to flip back and forth in the book.

Note: The recommendations given in this book are general, and not specific. So, please know yourself; if there's a food or herb or spice that you cannot consume or that makes you sick, DO NOT CONSUME IT! I have no way of knowing that about you from this side of my computer. Please apply your logic when choosing to explore recommendations. As my naturopathic doctor once told me after I requested a food allergy test, "Mona, you can get the test and it will tell you all sorts of things. The reality is, whether the test says it or not, if every time you eat potatoes you feel gross, then you have to stop eating potatoes, even if the test says you can eat them." Your body possesses so much wisdom. Ayurveda intends to open you to that inner knowing so you can guide yourself to health!

Note: Please know that I have not included any herbal recommendations in this book. I believe strongly that one needs an individual recommendation from a qualified practitioner before taking herbs, as they are potent medicine.

Once you've read through the book once, you can zoom in on the pieces that are most relevant for you. I include checklists and simple recommendations along the way. My hope is that you will find straightforward ways to begin stabilizing your own health using the three pillars and the ideas in this book.

Best wishes on your journey to health!

m xo

SECTION I:

OVERVIEW OF AYURVEDIC PRINCIPLES

Each patient carries his own doctor inside him.

—Norman Cousins

Introduction to Section I

Like all sciences, Ayurveda has unique perspectives. I like to think of these as "maps of the terrain," information that will help you to orient yourself in this living healing science so you can make the most of its teachings.

This section is to orient you to those perspectives. Once you have the content, the subsequent information on the three pillars of health will make more sense, and the bigger picture of health will be clearer.

In this section, we cover the language of Ayurveda, dimensions of being, three main causes of disease, and the power of choice.

CHAPTER 1

LANGUAGE OF AYURVEDA

Ayurveda describes everything in the world using a set language known as the qualities of nature, or the *gunas* in Sanskrit. Other translations of the Sanskrit word *guna* include "characteristic" or "attribute." This means that as you learn about Ayurveda, you will hear these same words over and over; this is done on purpose. The intention is to establish a common and concrete language that we can all work with. We're trying to get on the same page. If you plan to use Ayurveda, it will be helpful to get to know the language. Once we figure out the language, Ayurveda becomes very straightforward.

Something I deeply appreciate about this language is that when you're looking at the world through the lens of the qualities, there's no judgment to the observations. The language allows us to take all layers of judgment, guilt, shame, and critical mindset right out of play. For example, check in with the temperature of your body: "Do you feel hot, or do you feel cold?" Neither response, hot or cold, is good or bad; they simply are. Maybe today you're feeling cold; maybe today you're feeling warm. It is what it is. This allows us to stick to self-observation without judgment or preference, which is really important in order to use Ayurveda effectively. By using a language that is inherently non-critical, we develop the capacity to observe ourselves in a way that is compassionate and very real. Already we're paving the road to health and healing!

Now let's talk about the qualities![4] The table below outlines the qualities in fixed sets known as "the pairs of opposites." Knowing which qualities are in which pair is very important in order to use them skilfully, as we will soon see (spoiler alert!).

	Continuum	Building & Nourishing	Reducing & Lightening
1	Weight	Heavy	Light
2	Intensity	Dull or Slow	Sharp or Penetrating
3	Temperature	Cold	Hot
4	Emollience	Oily or Unctuous	Dry
5	Texture	Smooth	Rough
6	Viscosity	Dense or Thick or Solid	Liquid or Diluted
7	Compressibility	Soft	Hard
8	Fluidity	Stable	Mobile
9	Density	Gross	Subtle
10	Adhesion	Cloudy	Clear
	Bonus 1		Spreading
	Bonus 2		Flesh Smelling

Why Pairs of Opposites?

Are you curious about why we have these pairs of opposites? There are a few reasons. One is because we recognize that the qualities in each pair of opposites are connected to each

---

4   From the *Ashtanga Hrdayam, Sutrasthana 1.18.*

other; specifically, one cannot exist without the other. My teacher Dr. Claudia Welch describes them as the "yin and yang of Ayurveda." You can't tell if something is light unless you compare it to something heavy. Further, the object that is light might become heavy compared to something else. For example, if I take my cat, who is 20 pounds, and I compare her to my dog, who is 60 pounds, then we would describe the cat as light. However, if I compare my cat to a piece of paper from my printer, now the cat is heavy. What is light and what is heavy depends on what it is being compared to.

The qualities are not about a fixed point; they are relative to our experience. All the qualities are relative to your own sense of balance within yourself. When you're working with the qualities and you check in, "Do I feel hot or cold today?" it's an internal check. Either you feel warmer than before, in which case you feel warm or hot, or you feel colder than before, in which case you feel cool or cold. All things are relative, or context-dependent. This is why, I believe, the most common saying in Ayurveda is "It depends." And there's even a third option: maybe you can't tell. This likely means you have found your balance point in the middle of the pair of opposites.

Another aspect of this is that what feels hot or warming for me, as someone who tends to run cold, might be different from someone else who runs hot because their starting point on the continuum is different than my starting point. Everyone's pendulum of balance is different. This is why one recommendation (or food, or exercise program, or daily routine, or educational approach, or anything!) does not work for everyone. We're all different in terms of which qualities we embody, and therefore different in what we need in order to find balance.

Maybe you noticed there are two qualities on the chart that do not have a continuum and do not have an opposite. Let's talk about those. One of the more interesting (and very curious) aspects of the qualities is that, like in any system, there are some exceptions to the rules. In this case, there are two qualities seen in the body-mind-behaviour without an "official" opposite (trust me, I tried for the entire six years I was in Ayurveda school to get someone to give me an opposite, or to agree to the ones I proposed, to no avail), and therefore no continuum. We'll cover these, like the others, and it will be interesting for you to contemplate if and where these qualities arise for you.

Each of us embodies all the pairs of opposites as well as the bonus qualities. As we move through life, some qualities will be balanced, and others will be out of balance. This balance and imbalance shifts moment to moment and is influenced by how we live: what we eat, how we eat, how we practice self-care (or lack of it), and the way we structure our daily routines and lifestyles.

Like Increases Like[5]

Understanding these pairs of opposites is important because this is how we're going to bring balance to your system. If you are on one end of the continuum, this means that the pendulum of balance has swung in one direction. In Ayurveda we learn that applying the same quality to itself increases that

5   From the *Ashtanga Hrdayam, Sutrasthana 1.14.1.*

quality. For example, imagine you're feeling warm, and I offer you a cup of hot tea and I wrap you in a blanket and I turn up the heat by 10 degrees. What's going to happen? It is 99.9% likely that you're going to get warmer—maybe even be too hot for your own comfort and well-being because **like increases like**.

Opposites Balance[6]

How about this scenario: Imagine you're feeling too warm, and I give you a cup of mint water, I open the window, turn on the fan to get a little breeze going, and invite you to take off your socks and your hat and coat. Then what happens? There's a good chance that you're going to cool down and feel better. Applying the opposite quality brings things back into the middle, back into balance.

These pairs of opposites are really important because they give us a language to express our felt experience, and then they also give us a way to bring balance to our systems.

The language of the qualities is powerful, given the scope and depth of what you can describe using these terms. In Ayurveda school we are asked to figure out which qualities are present in our food (diet), season, lifestyle, and environment so we can balance all these aspects of our lives in order to promote health and well-being.

The next section describes what these qualities look like, so you can begin to recognize them.

---

6   From the *Ashtanga Hrdayam, Sutrasthana 1.14.1.*

A quick word about food: According to Ayurveda, the food we eat every day (of all the things we do daily) has the greatest impact on our health. In the sections below, I include information on the qualities of foods in their natural states. Each food has innate qualities, and yet these qualities can be changed based on how you prepare the food. The example my teacher Dr. Rosy gives is broccoli. There is a difference between the quality of raw broccoli, steamed broccoli, and broccoli sautéed in oil with spices. Same food, different qualities based on the preparation of the food. The lists below are not exhaustive, yet hopefully they're enough to get you started and pique your curiosity about this aspect of food.

A. WEIGHT—HEAVY

Environment / Nature

In nature, the heavy quality is related to the earth element. Earth is the heaviest of the five elements in Vedic Science. The dictionary defines *heavy* as "of great weight; difficult to lift or move" and "needing much physical effort."[7]

We find heaviness in the mountains, the ocean (Have you carried a 10L bottle of water? Can you imagine the weight of an ocean?), gravity, and soil. Elephants, trucks, buildings, bowling balls, metals, and trains are all heavy.

In the weather, heaviness manifests as wet snow (If you've ever shovelled it, you know how heavy this is!),

7 "Heavy," Google, accessed March 2018, https://www.google.ca/search?q=Dictionary.

mud, big rainfalls, and dense clouds (often described as a "heavy sky").

Body

In the body, we see heavy bones, heavy muscles, and a larger frame or skeleton. If there is an excess of the heavy quality, the body becomes overweight. Foods that have the heavy quality are very nourishing, which means they are excellent for building tissues in the body. Culturally, we tend to think that being heavy or overweight is "bad." We add a value judgment that is not inherently there, and we miss the other aspect, which is that nourishment is necessary. We want to cultivate enough heaviness that we're feeling nourished but not so much that we end up with excess. We are looking for our balance point even within the one quality.

Heaviness can manifest in a deep voice. Folks who embody heaviness feel grounded, centered, and stable. This is neat because stability is one of the other qualities on our list. We will see that sometimes the qualities work together and are not mutually exclusive. There is definitely interconnection between the different qualities.

The heavy quality manifests as slow digestion or slow metabolism, which means it takes a long time for food to digest. Slow digestion also happens if you eat too much heavy food, regardless of the nature of your digestion.

Mind and Emotions

We need enough of the heavy quality in order to fall asleep at night, which is super important, as sleep is one of Ayurveda's three pillars of health. It also manifests as deep thoughts. Where there's excess heaviness in the mind, one might feel tired, depressed, or like the world is too heavy. As the expression goes, "Carrying the weight of the world on our shoulders."

Foods

Foods that are heavy include meat (especially beef and pork), milk and cheese (most dairy products), oils, figs, peaches, almonds, pistachios, walnuts, apricots, dates, potatoes, sweet potatoes, and wheat. At its extreme is the deep-fried cheesesteak hoagie, which I suspect is the heaviest food ever created. The heavy quality is what makes these foods more challenging to digest, and also what makes them so satisfying and grounding.

B. WEIGHT—LIGHT

If we go to the opposite end of the continuum, we work with the **LIGHT** quality.

Environment / Nature

In nature, the light quality is related to the fire, air, and ether elements. This means that not only does lightness manifest as part of weight, but due to its connection to the fire element, also as sunshine and brightness.

The dictionary defines *light* in two broad categories— one with respect to sight (illumination) and the other with respect to weight. In terms of weight, which is what Ayurveda is describing, *light* means: "of little weight;

easy to lift" and "requiring little mental effort; not profound or serious."[8]

We find lightness in sand, rainbows, flowers, birds, feathers, paper, hummingbirds, and flies.

In the weather, lightness manifests as sunshine, wind, fluffy snow (which is a big difference from wet snow!), sprinkling rain, and in fast-moving clouds.

Body

In the body, this quality manifests as a light or thin frame or a slim build. In the realm of too much or excess lightness of the bone tissue, we see osteopenia and osteoporosis, referred to in the medical community as "light bones." Emaciation is a sign of excess light *guna*. We might also see fair or shiny skin or bright eyes. The Ayurvedic texts describe bright-light intolerance as an expression of excess light *guna*.

Those who have a lot of lightness tend to have challenges with sleep because they don't have enough of the heavy quality to settle in and sleep through the night. So we might notice lightness through scanty sleep or bouts of insomnia.

Mind and Emotions

A sense of lightness in the *mind* allows us to be alert and attentive. Too much lightness in the mind creates a feeling of being spacey, ungrounded, unstable, insecure, fearful, or anxious.

---

8 "Light," Google, accessed March 2018, https://www.google.ca/search?q=Dictionary.

Foods

Foods that are light include goat milk, boiled rice, rice flour, barley, quinoa, black pepper, and broths.

C. INTENSITY—DULL or SLOW

Environment / Nature

In nature, the dull or slow quality is related to the water element. Water is heavy, and things that are heavy move more slowly. I find it easier to recognize the slow quality—turtles, snails, and sloths. It is also found in the movement of tectonic plates (the continental plates), which move so slowly we don't even notice. Socks, blankets, Play-Doh, round buttons, and yoga bolsters are all dull—not in the sense of being boring, but in the sense of not having sharpness to them.

The dictionary defines *dull* as "less intense" and "lacking brightness, vividness, or sheen."[9] It defines *slow* as "not quick or fast" and "lasting or taking a long time."[10]

In the weather, slow manifests as long, never-ending days or a slow-moving storm. Dullness shows up as gloomy, cloudy, and foggy.

I feel like the slow quality needs cultivation in our culture because people are moving too fast. In Vedic speak, we

---

9 "Dull," Google, accessed March 2018, https://www.google.ca/search?q=Dictionary.

10 "Slow," Google, accessed March 2018, https://www.google.ca/search?q=Dictionary.

refer to this as being *"rajasic."* There is so much speediness, movement, and rushing around—go, go, go—which has consequences to our nervous system! With this in mind, I work with the slow quality a lot in my Ayurvedic practice.

Body

Physically, this quality manifests as being slow in action for folks who walk, talk, and digest slowly. There is dullness in the voice, skin, or eyes. They tend to have an attitude or a demeanour that is relaxed, calm, and quiet. Silence is attributed to the slow quality.

Mind and Emotions

The mind needs to be able to slow down, to unwind in order to settle into sleep, so this quality is very useful here. Some of us process emotions and thoughts more slowly. I know that I need more time to fully understand, digest, and integrate ideas. I'm not "quick on my feet" that way. Some have more dullness in the mind.

Foods

Foods that are dull or slow include beef and milk.

D. INTENSITY—SHARP or PENETRATING

If we go to the opposite end of the continuum, we work with the **SHARP and PENETRATING** quality. An object's ability to penetrate is a result of its sharp quality.

Environment / Nature

In nature, the sharp and penetrating quality is related to the fire element.

The dictionary defines *sharp* as "having an edge or point that is able to cut or pierce something" and "sudden and marked" and "precisely."[11] *Penetrating* is "able to make a way through or into something" and "succeed in understanding or gaining insight into."[12]

We find sharpness in a lion's roar, a circling hawk's call, sea urchins, the peaks of mountains, sharp turns on roads, swords, knives, and teeth. I also think of those sounds that cut right through you, penetrating to the depths of your being. This one is different for everyone—maybe it's fingernails on a chalkboard or a child throwing a tantrum.

In the weather, sharpness manifests as brisk wind, quick changes in weather patterns (was sunny and bright then quickly it is dark and stormy), lightning and thunder, or freezing rain—especially when the bits of ice hit your

---

11   "Sharp," Google, accessed March 2018, https://www.google.ca /search?q=Dictionary.

12   "Penetrating," Google, accessed March 2018, https://www.goog le.ca/search?q=Dictionary.

face! It also shows up as the warm sun penetrating your skin, or the damp penetrating your bones.

Body

In terms of physical features, we see a tapering chin, sharp teeth, distinct eyes, a pointed nose, or a heart-shaped face. Sharpness in the digestion leads to strong hunger. Where the digestion is too sharp (excessive), ulcers happen.

Mind and Emotions

Emotionally, sharpness is anger, rage, resentment, shame, and guilt. That said, sometimes guilt can feel dull too. It depends on the person.

In the mind, sharpness manifests as a strong memory, and strength in terms of understanding, comprehension, concentration, and learning. Think of avid students who have a strong hunger for knowledge, experience, and life—they go deep into the material (penetrating). When taken to the extreme, this attempt to feed the fire of the mind, beyond the body's ability to sustain it, leads to burnout.

Foods

Foods that are sharp or intense include onions, black pepper, ginger, garlic, and cayenne.

E. TEMPERATURE—COLD

Environment / Nature

In nature, the cold quality is related to the water and air elements.

Cold is defined as "of or at a low or relatively low temperature, especially when compared with the human body" and "lacking affection or warmth of feeling; unemotional."[13]

The cold quality is found in ice, sub-zero temperatures, raw foods, and dairy products.

In the weather, cold manifests when the temperature is below zero (I live in Canada, where zero degrees Celsius is freezing!) and in ice, snow, freezing rain, and fall and winter seasons. There are also cool breezes, which are a sweet relief in the summer.

Body

If we embody the cold quality, we are likely to have cold hands or feet, muscle stiffness, and clammy skin. Our digestion slows down too. Numbness comes from too much cold quality, which is why people put ice on their body to numb that area. Too much cold quality impairs the circulation and flow of fluid and heat in the body. Catching a cold is too much of the cold quality.

---

13   "Cold," Google, accessed March 2018, https://www.google.ca/search?q=Dictionary.

Mind and Emotions

Coldness manifests as insensitivity—as in the expression "that person is very cold." Unconsciousness, which is a lack of presence or strong numbness, is cold. Fear and insecurity are also connected to the cold quality.

Foods

Foods that are cold include milk, *ghee* (clarified butter), goat milk, cucumbers, limes, melons, grapes, coconuts, apples, basmati rice, cumin, coriander/cilantro, and fennel.

F. TEMPERATURE—HOT

If we go to the opposite end of the continuum, we work with the **HOT** quality.

Environment / Nature

In nature, the hot quality is related to the fire element.

Hot is defined as "having a high degree of heat or a high temperature."[14]

We find heat in fire, the desert, hot springs, friction, ovens, irons, cooked foods, spicy foods, and warm drinks.

In the weather, heat manifests as heat waves, warm winds, sunshine, and summertime.

---

14   "Hot," Google, accessed March 2018, https://www.google.ca/search?q=Dictionary.

Body

The most obvious is a warm body temperature—some people just run hot or are referred to as "warm-blooded." Gray hair and baldness are considered signs of heat in the head, where heat burns the colour out of the hair or burns the roots of the hair and the hair falls out, respectively. So where people are gray or balding, that's seen as excess heat. It also manifests as a strong appetite, digestive fire, absorption, and circulation.

Mind and Emotions

When there's an excess of heat, people become irritated, angry, impatient, and enraged. They might also express passion.

Foods

Foods that are hot include beef, venison, onions, garlic, ginger, chillies, sesame, mustard (and seeds), flax, hing/asafoetida, cinnamon, and alcohol (except for beer).

G. EMOLLIENCE—OILY or UNCTUOUS

Environment / Nature

The oily quality is associated with the water element. The dictionary defines *oily* as "containing oil."[15] It is found a lot in nature—many plants, nuts, and seeds contain oil, which we extract in order to consume it. Examples include essential oils (from plants like lavender, tea tree,

---

15   "Oily," Google, accessed March 2018, https://www.google.ca/search?q=Dictionary.

basil, cedar, etc.) and cooking oils (avocado, grapeseed, coconut, sesame, almond, olive, etc.). We also find oil in machinery, as it serves a lubricating function. My family owns a garage, and the amount of oil it takes to turn everyone's car into "a finely oiled machine" is wild!

A description of *oily weather*, as described by my best friend, Veronica, includes "Slightly warm, slightly greasy-feeling, damp. When you walk outside, your skin gets that slimy feeling." I think of it as connected to spring—moist and heavy.

Body

The oily quality is seen in the skin, hair, and feces. Another manifestation is well-lubricated joints. This means joints that don't snap, crackle, and pop. The "Rice Krispies" in the joints are actually an indication of dryness in the body, which is the opposite quality of oily. Those with oily as a quality have ample moisture in their bodies and have a smoothness about them—in body and even in demeanour.

Mind and Emotions

The oily quality is connected to relaxation, compassion, and love. I find this a sweet manifestation of a quality. 🖤

Foods

Foods that are oily include oils, beef, venison, fish, milk, yogurt, *ghee*, coconuts, almonds, and walnuts.

H. EMOLLIENCE—DRY

If we go to the opposite end of the continuum, we work with the **DRY** quality.

Environment / Nature

In nature, the dry quality is related to the air element.

Dry is defined as "free from moisture or liquid; not wet or moist."[16] We see dryness in deserts, sand and sandpaper, crackers, and cereals (flakes, puffs, etc.). Some grains like millet and buckwheat are drying, and even green veggies have a drying effect in the body, causing constipation. Many cleanses and cleansing foods are drying to the body.

In the weather, there are dry seasons when all the moisture disappears (dries up). Here in Ontario, Canada, we see dryness in the fall for sure, then sometimes in the summer (can be hot and dry), and sometimes in the winter (very cold and dry). The latter two are variable, since sometimes our summers are warm and moist; the same is true with winter. Where there is heat, there is evaporation, which results in dryness.

Body

Dryness shows in the body in our skin, hair, lips, and tongue—we feel the dryness as the moisture disappears. It is present in

---

16   "Dry," Google, accessed March 2018, https://www.google.ca/search?q=Dictionary.

a hoarse voice and coughing. Dryness also manifests as dehydration, constipation, and pain in the body.

Mind and Emotions

In the emotions and mind, dryness is connected to fear, nervousness, anxiety, and especially loneliness. I also see it in a "dry" sense of humour.

Foods

Foods that are dry include honey, barley, corn, buckwheat, millet, rice cakes, flakes (like cereal), crackers, and unsoaked chia seeds (have you noticed how much liquid these can absorb?).

I. TEXTURE—SMOOTH

Environment / Nature

The smooth quality is related to the water element. The dictionary defines *smooth* as "having an even and regular surface or consistency; free from perceptible projections, lumps, or indentations" and "without harshness or bitterness."[17]

In life, sometimes things are smooth and flow with ease, and other times they are rough. I think everyone has realized this contrast at some point in his or her life. Along these lines, I also think of "smooth transitions" as being seamless, calm, and straightforward.

---

17 "Smooth," Google, accessed March 2018, https://www.google.ca /search?q=Dictionary.

We see and experience this quality in smooth peanut butter, a snail trail, the surface of a rock eroded by the water, flat surfaces (a smooth road, trail, and ride), and slippery surfaces like an ice rink.

In terms of the weather, we have smooth sailing, calm waters, and calm skies. My friend Veronica describes it as "one of those days where the clouds in the sky are smooth and the air is not too warm and not too cold. The air is humid, but not unpleasantly so." And my sister Maggie went with "the pale blue or pearly grey days where the sky and water look the same."

Body

The manifestations are present in the skin (including lips!), hair, nails, organs, and joints. Those who have a lot of smooth quality are flexible because they move smoothly from one direction to the next. They transition with ease, so changes in direction are smooth. Those who don't have smoothness, who embody roughness instead, will find it hard to move in a lot of different directions and in a lot of different ways—transitions will challenge them.

Mind and Emotions

Flexibility can also be a quality of a smooth mind—flexible in thoughts and ideas and beliefs. We'll also see a calm nature and gentle mind in those who are smooth.

Foods

Foods that are smooth include most dairy, especially milk and *ghee*.

J. TEXTURE—ROUGH

If we go to the opposite end of the continuum, we work with the **ROUGH** quality.

Environment / Nature

The rough quality is related to the air element. It is defined as "having an uneven or irregular surface; not smooth or level" and "not gentle."[18] We see it in bumps in the road and rocks, the seams of our clothing, materials like corrugated cardboard and corduroy, sandpaper, transitions that are challenging, as well as difficult conversations.

In the weather, extreme temperatures (whether hot or cold) and extreme manifestations of weather patterns (water and waves, rain, snow, wind, storms, hail) are rough.

Body

Here we see cracked skin, nails, hands, feet, teeth, hair, cracking joints, and constipation. It manifests similarly to the dry quality, as there is a connection between the dry and rough qualities. I embody a lot of the dry quality, and I noticed that when my skin gets dry, it also feels rough.

Mind and Emotions

I am aware as I write this section that the qualities are in the "eye of the beholder" or the "experience of the experiencer."

18   "Rough," Google, accessed March 2018, https://www.google.ca /search?q=Dictionary.

For myself, there are some emotions that are "rougher" for me to experience, like shame, grief, and hurt. I know other people who find anger is what challenges them. We're all different in our perception of what is rough; this is true for every quality.

Rough in the mind for me is "the straw that breaks the camel's back," that point of "I just can't do this anymore," or "I just cannot handle one more challenge." At times, I also notice that my thoughts don't always flow in a smooth and coherent way—they are jagged and all over the place. It's like the container of my mind gets rough.

Foods

Foods that are rough include raw veggies, dry salad, dry cereal, rice cakes, and crackers.

K. VISCOSITY—DENSE or THICK or SOLID

Environment / Nature

The dense quality belongs to the earth element. It is also sometimes referred to as "thick." In scientific terms, *density* refers to "mass per cubic inch."[19] It's not about how heavy something is, although dense things tend to also be heavy.

We see density and thickness in concrete, large objects (rocks, buildings, mountains), rainforests (thick plant covering), metals (the densest being osmium), and neutron stars, which are apparently the densest objects in

---

19 "Dense," Google, accessed March 2018, https://www.google.ca /search?q=Dictionary.

the universe. I am also reminded of molasses, honey, and roast beef—thick, dense foods.

In terms of the weather, we have thick fog and clouds, dense smog, and humidity.

Body

The manifestations of dense and thick are seen in the skin, hair, nails, and feces (bowel movements that clog tend to be dense and thick). Think of a person with compact and condensed tissues. A useful stereotype here is the classic image of football players and rugby players—how dense and thick their biology is. In these body types, we often see a limitation in the range of motion because there is so much dense tissue that the joints find compression quickly. Firm, solid, and strong muscles are dense.

Mind and Emotions

This quality promotes a feeling of groundedness. It can also manifest as thick-headedness, foggy brain/thinking, or a lack of space, movement, or flexibility in the mind.

Foods

Foods that are dense or thick include milk, yogurt, cheese, meat, molasses, and bananas.

L. VISCOSITY—LIQUID or DILUTED

If we go to the opposite end of the continuum, we work with the **LIQUID** quality.

Environment / Nature

In nature, the liquid quality is related to the water element. The dictionary defines *liquid* as "a substance that flows freely but is of constant volume."[20] From the Ayurvedic perspective, this involves the idea of dilution, which is the change of a dense and thick material to one that is more liquid or diluted. According to the dictionary, *dilution* is defined as "the action of making something weaker in force, content, or value,"[21] reducing concentration, reducing thickness. There is more space between the molecules or component pieces.

We see liquid everywhere—water, soda, tea, coffee, rivers, lakes, and oceans.

In the weather, look for water—rain, snow, steam, humidity, and clouds.

Body

The human body is very liquid. Babies are over 90% water, and adults are closer to 70% water. We embody liquid in sweat, urine, thirst, salivation, plasma, and mucous. Where there's

---

20   "Liquid," Google, accessed March 2018, https://www.google.ca /search?q=Dictionary.

21   "Dilution," Google, accessed March 2018, https://www.google.ca /search?q=Dictionary.

excess liquid, it can pool or accumulate, which causes a variety of issues like edema and congestion (mucous buildup) in the chest, sinuses, throat, and head.

Mind and Emotions

Emotions are fluid by their very nature in that they arise, exist, and dissolve. With a connection to the water element, we see liquidity in our tears and sorrow.

In the mind, I see both liquid and diluted. The liquid aspect manifests as the flow of thoughts, ideas, and inspirations, and the chatter of my ego. The diluted aspect shows up when I can't focus on something.

Foods

Foods that are liquid or diluted include water, juice, milk, watermelons, cantaloupes, cucumbers, and juicy fresh fruits.

M. COMPRESSIBILITY—SOFT

Environment / Nature

The soft quality belongs to the water element. I love the dictionary's definition of *soft*: "easy to mold, cut, compress or fold." Also "a pleasing quality that involves a subtle effect or contrast rather than a sharp definition."[22]

Softness is found in kitten and bunny fur, cashmere, velvet, feathers, flower petals, marshmallows, pudding, and mud.

---

22 "Soft," Google, accessed March 2018, https://www.google.ca/search?q=Dictionary.

In terms of the weather, I found many articles online about how "soft" often translates to "mild" or "calm" when referring to the weather. We also see it in soft snow, soft rainfalls, and soft fluffy clouds.

Body

The soft quality presents in the skin, hair, nails, tissues, and mucous (considered the softest of the body's fluids). One of the classical texts says, "a pleasing look," which I did not understand until reading the dictionary definition around subtle contrasts versus sharp—soft features in the shape of one's face, body, eyes, and being.

Mind and Emotions

This quality emphasizes forgiveness, love, compassion, kindness, and tenderness. I also consider softness in the mind a form of malleability and flexibility, or in other words, a lack of rigidity and fixed mind.

Foods

Foods that are soft include milk, *ghee*, soups, and oils.

N. COMPRESSIBILITY—HARD

If we go to the opposite end of the continuum, we work with the **HARD** quality.

Environment / Nature

In nature, the hard quality is related to the earth element. According to the dictionary, *hard* is defined as "resistant to pressure; not easily broken, bent, or pierced" and "requiring a great deal of endurance or effort."[23]

The hardest naturally occurring substance on earth is the diamond. There are many other hard substances, some natural and some engineered. These include Kevlar, spider's silk, silicon carbide (used to make tanks), bedrock, cobblestone, and sandstone.

In the weather, look for challenging or extreme weather of any type—ice, storms of all types (ice, wind, rain), heat, drought, etc.

Body

Physically, this quality manifests as hard muscles, bones, nails, and teeth. It is interesting because I think people move away from hardness, and yet there are some tissues that are healthiest when they are hard—like the bones, nails, and teeth. You might also see calluses on the hands and feet, which can come from hard work. Hardness is connected to

---

23   "Hard," Google, accessed March 2018, https://www.google.ca/search?q=Dictionary.

strength, hence why we might see this in the muscle tissue as well.

Mind and Emotions

What is hard in terms of emotions varies from person to person. Which are the emotions that are the most challenging, the hardest for you to be with and process? I observe that grief is hard for most people. This quality is also connected with insensitivity, rigidity, selfishness, and callousness.

I often listen to Pema Chödrön's audiobooks, and she says, "The opposite of a flexible mind would be a rigid [hard] one."[24] Hardness can be fixed, firm, set, and without movement.

Foods

Foods that are hard include nuts (unless soaked), pretzels, and raw veggies.

O. FLUIDITY—STABLE

Environment / Nature

The stable quality belongs to the earth element. This goes well with the dictionary definition of stability as "not likely to give way or overturn; firmly fixed" and "not likely to change or fail; firmly established."[25] Stability manifests in nature through consistent rhythms and patterns (cycles), mountains, rocks, and earth (solid ground).

---

24   Pema Chödrön, *Getting Unstuck* (Sounds True, 2005).

25   "Stable," Google, accessed March 2018, https://www.google.ca /search?q=Dictionary.

In terms of the weather, stability manifests as consistency within a season or seasonal pattern. Here in Canada we would say a warm summer, windy fall, snowy winter, and rainy spring. These are the patterns we expect, and the patterns that make sense for us. Stability in weather happens when a season expresses as expected (e.g., no snow in June!).

Body

Stability is found in solid joints, bones, and body. People who have a lot of stability have fewer injuries and illnesses. Their high embodiment of stability means their body is very resilient.

Mind and Emotions

It is the ability to sit quietly, to sleep well, and to do nothing. Without enough stability, there can be no healing or change that takes place in the body. Lasting change only happens when there is solid ground on which those changes can take hold. This is why stability is a quality I often try to cultivate for myself and for my students.

For me, stability of the heart-mind is mental-emotional stability. This feels like fewer mood swings and fewer unpredictable reactions. The Yogic system is designed to cultivate *sattva* (harmony and balance in the mind), and I intend to maintain a connection to *sattva* even when my day is a roller coaster. This takes way less energy than riding the swing of the pendulum between *rajas* (agitation of the heart-mind) and *tamas* (dulling or numbing out). For more details on these concepts of the mind, keep reading. ☺

Foods

Foods that are stable include meat (beef in particular), wheat, nuts, and root vegetables.

P. FLUIDITY—MOBILE

If we go to the opposite end of the continuum, we work with the **MOBILE** quality.

Environment / Nature

In nature, the mobile quality is related to the air element; think of wind. According to the dictionary, *mobile* is defined as "able to move or be moved freely or easily."[26] Other language that infers the mobile *guna* includes *transformation, change, active, variable, unstable, restless,* and *erratic.* What is interesting is how the two opposite qualities need each other: in order to have lasting change, there has to be enough stability to hold the transformation. It really is about finding balance and not being extreme.

Mobility is found everywhere: the movement of the planets in our solar system, phases of the moon, growth cycles, wind blowing, tide coming in (and going back out), running, walking, moving, jumping, dancing, evolving, and breathing (inhale into exhale, exhale into inhale).

In the weather, mobility is high during the seasonal changes, when we're switching from one season to

---

26   "Mobile," Google, accessed March 2018, https://www.google.ca /search?q=Dictionary.

another. Another way the mobile quality shows up in the weather is when something is unseasonable, as in when there is a variation in the seasonal norm (e.g., snow in June). And let's not forget hurricanes and tornadoes!

Body

This quality manifests in movement of all sorts. Think of people who talk a lot and move their hands while talking. When the mobile quality increases significantly, we begin to see instability or erratic movements (instead of smooth and fluid). Hypermobility is instability in the joints, which means dislocations. Other manifestations include tremors, shakiness, seizures, restless eyes (like someone who cannot make eye contact or focus on one point), moving eyebrows, and restless leg syndrome. Folks with a lot of mobility are constantly walking, talking, traveling, and multitasking.

Mind and Emotions

Mobility in the emotional body is experiencing the flow of emotion as well as a change in the emotions. Mobile minds have dreams, scattered dreams, a lot of thoughts, thoughts all over the place, restlessness, insecurity, anxiety, and erratic behaviour. Mental instability includes mood swings, manic depression, and bipolar disorder.

Foods

Foods that are mobile include carbonated beverages and caffeinated beverages.

Q. DENSITY—GROSS

Environment / Nature

The gross quality, also described as big and obvious, relates to the earth element. The dictionary describes *gross* as "general or large-scale; not fine or detailed" and "very obvious; blatant."[27] *Obvious* is described as "easily perceived or understood; clear, self-evident, or apparent."[28] *Big* is described as "of considerable size, extent, or intensity."[29]

We see this quality in the Rocky Mountains, the Grand Canyon, the Great Barrier Reef, and the trees in Stanley Park in British Columbia. (If you're curious, Google "photos of Stanley Park, BC, trees.") Houses, cars, elephants, whales, and hippos are all things (and beings) that are big in size.

In terms of the weather, the gross quality shows up in the bigger weather patterns like storms that move across the globe or a high-rated earthquake. Also, in the obvious—when it's raining, it's raining. If it's warm, it's warm. When it's cold, it's cold.

---

27 "Gross," Google, accessed March 2018, https://www.google.ca /search?q=Dictionary.

28 "Obvious," Google, accessed March 2018, https://www.google.ca /search?q=Dictionary.

29 "Big," Google, accessed March 2018, https://www.google.ca/sear ch?q=Dictionary.

Body

Grossness manifests as things that are large in size—frame (very tall or stout), bones, hands, feet, nose, and eyes. They are all things that are gross, big, and obvious. Obesity is an excess of the big quality.

Mind and Emotions

This quality means that a person is not able to hide how they feel—like the saying that a person "has no poker face." People feel how they feel, and it is obvious, or written all over them.

They might also feel their emotions more because they are so obvious. Another interpretation is that the emotions might feel "big" to them. This can also manifest as a big or very dramatic personality.

Foods

Foods that are gross, obvious, or big include wheat, meat, and dairy.

R. DENSITY—SUBTLE or MINUTE

If we go to the opposite end of the continuum, we work with the **SUBTLE** quality.

Environment / Nature

In nature, the subtle quality is related to the ether element. Depending on the text, sometimes also the air element. These aren't seen with the naked eye, only inferred. According to the dictionary, subtle is defined as "so delicate or precise as to be difficult to analyze or describe" and "understated."[30] Another translation for the Sanskrit of this word is *minute* as in "extremely small."

The subtle quality is the twinkle in someone's eye, the fine threads of a silk blouse, the beating of a hummingbird's wings, the details of a feather, the gradual blooming of a flower, and fleas.

In the weather, subtlety is when we're not sure what we're seeing, like a fine mist on the water. Or when we wonder, *Is that rain outside?* It is also micro-climates and small weather patterns (it's raining here but not across the street) and small differences in light at different times of day.

Body

Subtlety manifests as goose bumps, twitches, and fine tremors. Energy is very subtle, as not everyone can see it.

One of the tools commonly used in Ayurveda is yoga. Yoga is a science of self-realization, which means you get to know and understand yourself. It uses many tools that allow us to understand ourselves better, and some of these tools are quite subtle—like postures, breath work, meditation, *mantra* (chanting sacred sounds), *mudras* (sacred gestures).

Mind and Emotions

A couple of other mental-emotional manifestations of subtlety can be spaciness, anxiety, and insecurity. I believe there is a connection of subtlety to awareness too—sometimes what we

---

30   "Subtle," Google, accessed March 2018, https://www.google.ca /search?q=Dictionary.

are experiencing is so subtle that it is under our level of awareness. For example, I had no idea how anxious and angry I was (for decades) until life circumstances made it obvious. Interestingly, I didn't get more angry or anxious, I simply wasn't aware, or we could say that it was not obvious to me that I felt this way.

Foods

Foods that are subtle or minute include salt, sugar, caffeine, *ghee*, and alcohol.

S. ADHESION—CLOUDY

Environment / Nature

The cloudy quality, also described as sticky and slimy, is related to the water element. It reminds me of mud, the mixture of water and earth together.

The dictionary describes *cloudy* as "not transparent or clear" and "covered with or characterized by clouds."[31] *Sticky* is described as "tending or designed to stick to things on contact,"[32] and *slimy* is "covered by or having the feel or consistency of slime."[33]

---

31 "Cloudy," Google, accessed March 2018, https://www.google.ca /search?q=Dictionary.

32 "Sticky," Google, accessed March 2018, https://www.google.ca /search?q=Dictionary.

33 "Slimy," Google, accessed March 2018, https://www.google.ca/se arch?q=Dictionary.

We see this quality in clouds and cloudy substances (like coconut water), slugs, fish, okra, and tree sap (sticky).

In terms of the weather, look for overcast skies and foggy or cloudy days. Notice if the earth is hard or muddy (mud is sticky). Also, when it's hot, damp, and muggy.

Body

It manifests in the body as mucous, which is cloudy, sticky, and slimy. Stickiness also refers to compact, firm joints: a joint that sticks together well, that has good cohesion, as opposed to a joint that dislocates. This quality promotes good cohesion in the body (sticks together) and manifests in someone who has a solid and firm structure (body).

Mind and Emotions

Cloudiness, in the mind and emotions, is connected to a lack of awareness and a lack of clarity, like seeing through rose-coloured glasses.

Those who have a lot of cloudy-sticky-slimy quality have great cohesion, including in relationships. Those who have a lot of sticky quality love to hug and become deeply attached in their relationships, even "stuck" on someone, for better or for worse.

Everyone needs enough of the sticky quality to retain memory. Each memory is an imprint that sticks in the mind—no sticky, no memory.

Foods

Foods that are cloudy, sticky, or slimy include okra, eggplant, soaked chia seeds, yogurt, condensed milk, and fish.

T. ADHESION—CLEAR

If we go to the opposite end of the continuum, we work with the **CLEAR** quality.

Environment / Nature

In nature, the clear quality is related to the air and ether elements, neither of which can be seen with the naked eye, only inferred. According to the dictionary, *clear* is defined as "transparent" and "easy to perceive, understand, or interpret."[34]

The clear quality is looking into the ocean and seeing right to the bottom to the coral and the fish. Think also of Saran Wrap, glass jars, sheer materials like lace, and eyeglasses.

In the weather, clear is found in a cloudless sky that allows us to see the brightness of the sun, moon, stars, and planets with our naked eyes.

Body

Clarity shows itself in the eyes, skin, tongue, and nasal passages when these are unobstructed—the whites of the eyes are

---

34 "Clear," Google, accessed March 2018, https://www.google.ca/search?q=Dictionary.

white, the skin is clear of pimples and breakouts, the tongue is not coated with a layer of slimy-sticky undigested metabolic waste (known in Sanskrit as *ama*, which we'll talk about more later in the book), and the nasal passages are free of mucous. My skin is also clear in the sense of being translucent; you can easily see my blood vessels and connective tissues. I joke with my doctor that I'm not pale, I'm "transparent."

A place we see clear a lot nowadays is through excessive cleansing—from anti-bacterial everything to being on a dietary cleanse all the time. I find it helpful to remember that cleansing is important, and yet, so is nourishment (read further to learn more about this very important first pillar of health!) if I want my body and mind to have the building blocks they need for health.

Mind and Emotions

The clear quality manifests in the mind as immediate under-standing (information is clear to a person); however, it can also manifest as forgetfulness. If you don't have enough sticky, you're not going to retain the information. Clear seeing is related to the yogic concept of reality, known in Sanskrit as *satya*. Yoga practice, generally speaking, helps us to clear our channels and disentangle ourselves from suffering.

The clear quality manifests in experiences of loneliness, emp-tiness, void, and isolation.

Foods

Foods that are clear include water, clear broth, and clear liquids.

U. SPREADING

This is the first BONUS quality, as I like to call them. It is one of the qualities that has no opposite and, therefore, no continuum. In my experience, these qualities are quite specific and have a lot of the fire element.

Environment / Nature

In nature, the spreading quality is related to the fire element. We know that, if left to its own devices, fire spreads. According to the dictionary, *spread* is defined as "open out (something) so as to extend its surface area, width, or length" and "extend over a large or increasing area."[35]

The spreading quality is seen in wildfires that extend and expand, sometimes out of control, as well as in the mint in my garden and a variety of other plants and greenery that expand and take over an area.

In the weather, storm fronts spread across an entire continent—the heat wave I experience in Canada is the result of a tropical storm last month in Puerto Rico.

Body

Spreading shows up in how the nutrition we consume doesn't just stay in our tummies but goes out to all cells and tissues of the body. We might also experience it in the skin, as in a spreading rash or itch. (Have you ever chased an itch? It

---

35   "Clear," Google, accessed March 2018, https://www.google.ca/search?q=Dictionary.

was one place, then it moves around, then you can feel it everywhere.)

Mind and Emotions

Those with the spreading quality might desire the spreading of their name, either by naming people or things after themselves or by seeking fame (seeing their name in large letters on a billboard or poster).

I have the spreading quality; however, mine manifests in how I work. When I take on a new project, especially something big, it starts with a pile of books, spreading to open books with bookmarks and a ton of sticky notes on the books and walls. Then I spread out all my resources (sometimes in many rooms, to my husband's dismay). As the project comes to a conclusion, everything comes back in on itself and gets put away, as if it never happened.

Foods

Foods that spread include hot, spicy foods.

V. FLESH SMELLING

This is the second BONUS quality. It is the other quality that has no opposite and, therefore, no continuum. In my experience, the bonus qualities are quite specific and connected to having a lot of the fire element.

Environment / Nature

In nature, the flesh smell is related to the fire element. There is no dictionary definition of this quality, and it is a specific attribute that connects to the physical body.

Body

Flesh smell is just that, the smell of one's body. Those of us who have this quality know it. Those who don't might not understand. It is often misinterpreted as body odour or something putrid or rotten smelling, yet this is not flesh smell. Body odour and putrid body smells are an indication that something is amiss in the body—whether it's that things are not digesting properly (more on that in the next section of the book) or that we have consumed something that was putrid to start with.

I have this quality, and when I get really warm on the inside, you can smell my flesh. It's not BO or stinky or dirty or anything like that. It's more musky actually.

Foods

Foods that induce the flesh smelling quality in those who have it include hot, spicy foods.

Conclusion to the Qualities

To work with Ayurveda in a skilful way, we benefit from learning the language of Ayurveda, which are the qualities of nature. We learn to see them and feel them in our own experience. This gives us feedback on what is happening inside and outside of our body-mind. Our body is always giving us information, and Ayurveda wants to help us understand its language so we know what it's trying to tell us.

Now we know that in order to bring balance to our system, we need to figure out which quality is out of balance and then apply the opposite quality. If your skin is dry, do an oil massage. If you're feeling cold, drink a cup of hot tea. If you feel heavy, go for a walk or watch a funny movie to lighten up.

This is, as you may have noticed, a lot of moving pieces to balance. Once you get the hang of it, though, it becomes really straightforward. Keep reading to get a better understanding of the map and the terrain. The picture becomes more and more *clear* as you go along.

Remember, you can come back and read this a few more times to help it *stick* in your memory.

How the Qualities Relate to Constitution (Dosha)

You might be surprised that I've spent a ton of time and pages so far writing about the qualities of nature, especially given that most resources, when talking about Ayurveda, approach it from the lens of the *doshas* (constitutions or organizing energies).

Now that we understand the language of the qualities, let's see how it relates to this concept of *dosha*. At a basic level, each constitution has its own qualities, based on the elements that make up the *dosha*. Below I outline which *dosha* is connected with which elements and which qualities. Notice how each *dosha* has different qualities.

Vata—*Air and Ether*

Vata dosha, or the organizing energy that is made up of the air and ether elements, has the following qualities: cold, light, dry, rough, subtle, mobile, and clear.[36]

Pitta—*Fire and Water*

Pitta dosha, or the organizing energy that is made up of the fire and water elements, has the following qualities: hot, sharp/penetrating, slightly oily, light, liquid, spreading, and flesh smelling.[37]

Kapha—*Water and Earth*

Kapha dosha, or the organizing energy that is made up of the water and earth elements, has the following qualities: heavy, slow/dull, cold, oily, smooth, soft, stable, obvious, and cloudy/sticky/slimy.[38]

As you can see, figuring out your constitution is more complex because it's not just a single quality but a group of qualities. Another layer is that each person has all three constitutions within them, as each of these organizing energies governs certain tissues and functions in the body. This is a lot of moving pieces, and it is no surprise that we can be challenged in figuring out all the pieces.

What I really appreciate about the language of the qualities is that even if you can't figure out your *dosha,* you can recognize

---

36   From the *Ashtanga Hrdayam, Sutrasthana 1.11.*

37   From the *Ashtanga Hrdayam, Sutrasthana 1.12.*

38   From the *Ashtanga Hrdayam, Sutrasthana 1.12.*

the predominant qualities in your being and use the pairs of opposites to create more balance in your life.

Section Conclusion

In the next chapter, I'm going to use this language of the qualities to guide you through our next map—the Ayurvedic and Yogic maps of the human being! It's very cool and continues to lay the groundwork to learn about the pillars of health.

CHAPTER 2

DIMENSIONS OF BEING

In the previous chapter we talked about the language of Ayurveda and how the qualities of nature allow us to describe our environment, world, and experience. In this chapter, we'll focus on the elements of being human.

Ayurveda considers the human being to be more than just a body. Human beings have a body; however, there are other layers, or aspects, that we need to pay attention to if we want deep and stable health for the long term. The holistic approach of Ayurveda comes through its view of the person as being more than a body. We see the human being as having five distinct *layers of being* wrapped around their spirit or soul:

1. **Physical Body:** our literal biology, the part of us made up of the food we eat and the tissues produced from that food.

2. **Energy Body:** the part of us made up of the essence of breath and the energy of our subatomic particles and their movements.

3. **Emotional Body:** the part of us with instincts, our fear response, our habit patterns, and our feelings and emotions.

4. **Wisdom Body:** the part of us that can "self-observe," that knows from deep inside, and our intuition.

5. **Bliss Body:** the part of us that is joyful for no reason other than being.

6. **Spirit/Soul:** the deepest essence of who we are, the reason we are here and have a body, the part of us that is inextricably intertwined with everyone and everything in existence.

We might be tempted to think of these layers as separate pieces, but they aren't. They are deeply interconnected. If anything, the layers meld into one another; they overlap. Each layer is deeply connected to the layers right next door, so the physical body is strongly connected to the energy, and the emotions are strongly connected to the mind. Ayurveda teaches us that the more subtle layers, like the mind and spirit, strongly influence the more obvious layers, like the body and energy. And the reverse is true, too: the body does affect the mind, and it takes longer for the information to pass from the outer layers to the inner layers, and very little time for the information to pass from the inner layers to the outer.

Within each of these layers, I view the human being as a series of channels, like the plumbing in your house. We have different channels for different things—like food, wastes, fluids, emotions, and thoughts. One way of describing health is to say that our channels (or you can think of them as pipes) are strong and clear, and things can flow freely—no clogs or backups, no rust or residue. When things flow freely through our channels, we feel healthy, strong, capable, and clear.

So let's talk through the layers of being, the different types of channels we have.

Physical Body

I refer to this layer as the "biology," very literally our anatomy and physiology (like in biology class). In Western culture, this is the aspect of the self that we most strongly identify with, as it is the most obvious one. And, fair enough, our physical body plays an important role in our health. It is also the container for our being—it's the vehicle we ride around in for our lifetime, and much like any vehicle, it requires regular care and maintenance.

We need to be aware of and pay attention to the body, its channels, and the messages it sends us. The section on nourishment (pillar 1) goes into detail about our biology. This section teaches you about the various channels and tissues and will help you learn the language of the body, what it is trying to tell you, and how to support and work with your biology (instead of against it, which totally happens).

Sense Organs

An important part of our biology, specifically mentioned in the definition of health, is the sense organs. Each sense organ is its own channel and allows information to flow either into your system or from your system out into the world.

Ayurveda recognizes two categories of sense organs.

The first are the *organs of knowledge*. These are the sense organs that bring information from the outside world into your awareness, which is how we get knowledge. These are the ears for hearing, the skin for receiving touch, the eyes for sight, the tongue for taste, and the nose for smell.

The second are the *organs of action*. Based on the information we take in (knowledge), often we want to respond outward into the world, and for this we take action. The organs of action are our vocal cords for speech, our hands for grasping, our feet for locomotion, the genitourinary system for urination and procreation, and the anus for elimination (defecation specifically).

The sense organs are very important because they relay information about our environment to the mind for processing. When we refer to environment, we mean outside your body, like, "It's cold outside. I need a hat," or "It's raining out. Where's my umbrella?" We also mean inside your body, too, like, "I'm hungry," or "My low back is achy." All of these internal cues are being sent through the nervous system, which transmits all the sensory data and information to the brain and mind for processing. From there, the mind processes, interprets, and decides on any actions that need to take place.

From the Ayurvedic view, if you are to clearly understand what is happening in your world, if you are going to make choices that lead you to optimal health, your sense organs have to be healthy, functional, and clear. Hence why Ayurveda recommends spending time every day caring for the sense organs. As you work your way through the book, notice how many recommendations include clearing, maintaining, and supporting the sense organs. If your sense organs are not clear, and the information you receive is not accurate, how are you supposed to make healthy choices? Your choices are only as sound as the information coming into your system.

Energy Body

The layer right next to our physical body is a subtler layer made up of *prana*. *Prana* is the Sanskrit word for "vital life force," and it is the energy that enlivens us. *Prana* is the subtle energy of the breath, and so sometimes this layer is called the "breath body."

This layer of our being is deeply connected to the physical body; we could say these layers share a seam. Some people call this energy body their "aura," which is part of it; however, the energy body isn't only surrounding our physical selves, it is intertwined with our biology. It's what gives the biology the energy to do what it does. The channels of *prana* run parallel to the channels of your biology. We feel like we have plenty of energy as long as the channels are clear and the energy can flow freely through the channels.

Have you ever felt like something wasn't quite right? Maybe you felt "off" and yet when you went to the doctor and got tested, nothing came up? Sometimes our imbalances are subtler than the biology, so it's handy to remember that you are more than your physical body. You have multiple layers, all of them affecting your health and well-being.

Emotional Body

Feelings and emotions ... if you're human, you have them. We all do. This is a fascinating layer to our existence, and it is not only our emotions, but all the old patterns that can trigger them too. My therapist explains that most of our default habit patterns get set from birth to age seven. These patterns, known as *samskaras* in Sanskrit, are stored in the emotional layer. Our patterns, the things we do without thinking, greatly affect our health—health-promoting patterns increase our health, and non-health-promoting patterns decrease our health.

Another piece to the puzzle of this layer is allowing things to flow through the channels. Anytime we suppress and repress our emotions, we create clogs in the channels, and this takes away from our overall health. The other end of this is over-flow—where there is a backlog of emotional energy—and once the gate is opened it flows fiercely. In Ayurveda we seek balance: not underflow, not overflow, balanced flow through all the channels.

Wisdom Body

Mind

In the West, we tend to think of the mind as the "brain." Ayurveda invites us to expand on this belief, and to understand that our ability to think and process information happens throughout the whole body. Awareness goes beyond one organ; it permeates our entire being. You could think of your whole body as being intelligent and able to give you infor-mation. The channels of the mind are all pervasive—they are connected to every aspect and layer of your being from the most obvious (biology) to the most subtle (spirit).

If we look at this from a physiological perspective, the tissues that make up the brain (our nerve cells) are found through-out the entire body, with groupings of these cells in the heart and in the gut (enteric nervous system). We have intelligence spread throughout our being, not just in our heads. This may be a new perspective for you, yet I invite you to try it on and see how this idea feels.

According to Ayurveda, there are multiple aspects to the mind:

- ✧ **Higher consciousness**, which allows us to watch ourselves and connects us to our intuition (quiet, calm, loving voice).

- ✧ **Ego**, which is our personality and the container for our likes and dislikes (louder voice).

- ✧ **Memory**, which stores all the information that passes through our field of awareness.

- ✧ **Sensory Mind**, which processes the information that comes in through the sense organs (which illustrates another connection between the layers).

I really appreciate how Ayurveda explains the complexity of our minds. This helps me to understand how it is more than an organ, and a more multidimensional concept.

When describing the mind and what is happening in the mind, Ayurveda uses a specific language (again). It is related to the qualities we already talked about but has its own words or descriptors.

Balanced Mind (sattva)

When the mind is balanced, it is described as being light, clear, stable, peaceful, and harmonious. In Sanskrit we call this *sattva*. Ayurveda teaches us that *sattva* is the nature of the mind, which means this *sattvic* state is accessible to everyone because it's our starting point (phew!). This is the mental state of contentment, peace, harmony, and even bliss. It is a very popular place. ☺ It is also the place of compassionate non-judgment, which is helpful for everyone.

That said, as we go through life, the pendulum of the mind can swing off of its balance point. When it swings, it tends to move either toward agitation or dullness. Let's explore these further.

Agitated Mind (rajas)

As the pendulum of the mind swings out of balance, on one end we have the state of mental agitation. In Sanskrit we call this *rajas*. The state of agitation is characterized by movement (mobility), heat, distraction, restlessness, and busyness. And when the pendulum swings really far in this direction, we might feel overwhelmed, anxious, or hyperactive, experience insomnia, and be unable to focus our attention on anything.

Before you start to think that agitation is a bad thing—hold your horses! There is a proper time and place for the movement of the mind, like when you are problem-solving, trying to get work done, or driving your car. Where we get into trouble is when the mind becomes active and cannot get back to its clear, stable, and calm state of balance. Sometimes our mind gets stuck in "agitation mode." An example is worrying: when you keep playing scenarios over and over again in your mind and trying to come up with what you'll say or what you'll do, like a hamster running in the wheel. The wheel doesn't go anywhere, but wow that hamster gets tired. This type of mental overwork definitely affects health.

Dull Mind (tamas)

When the pendulum swings in the opposite direction of agitation, we land in dullness. In Sanskrit we call this *tamas*. This state of mind is described as heavy, dull, dark, and inert. We might feel tired, lethargic, exhausted, or down. At its extreme we might experience depression or addiction (stuck in a rut of thought or behaviour).

Again, before you start thinking that dullness is a bad thing— hang on! There is a proper time and place for the dullness of the mind, like when it's time for rest, sleep, or healing. Have you ever noticed your mind gets dull when you catch a cold? It's to help you rest and recover! Where we get into trouble is when the mind becomes dull and cannot get back to its clear, light, and calm state of balance. Sometimes our mind gets stuck in "dullness mode," like depression or addiction.

It's not that dullness or agitation are bad states, it's the getting stuck on either end, losing the flow through the channels of the mind, that causes health issues. When we discussed the qualities of nature, we talked about how the language lets us approach life from a place of non-judgment. We can say the same about the language that describes the mind.

Did you notice how the descriptions of the mind include emotions? Balanced mind is loving, joyful, and contented. Agitated mind is anxious, fearful, and angry. Dull mind is sad, shameful, and depressed. Our emotional layer of being and its channels are deeply interconnected with the channels and experiences of the mind.

The qualities of the mind are influenced by the qualities of our food, lifestyle, seasons, stage of life, and environment. This book gives you an opportunity to explore how to work with your mind using these tools. For more on how to use food to cultivate a balanced mind, check out my friend Kate O'Donnell's book *Everyday Ayurveda Cooking for a Calm, Clear Mind: 100 Simple Sattvic Recipes*.

We're all born with the mind in a state of balance and then through life, living, and experience, the mind moves off of its center of harmony and balance. When it does, it moves in one of two directions: agitation or dullness. Sometimes these movements are very subtle, and sometimes these movements are very obvious. Either way, Ayurveda can help you bring more balance to your mind so you can feel healthier and more stable.

Bliss Body

This layer is the layer closest to the spirit or essence of our being, and its proximity and connection to our deepest essence is why it is blissful and joyful.

Spirit/Soul

To begin, a disclaimer: The last thing I am interested in is selling you a belief system. I am very aware that many people have a lot of opinions on spirit, soul, God, etc. Please feel free to substitute the words I'm using for words that work better for you.

I'm going to speak a little bit more generally about soul, and you might have a very different idea or interpretation of what that is and what that means to you. Keep the interpretation that resonates with you. I'm going to share my understanding of what I've learned about the Vedic view.

In the Vedic teachings, where Ayurveda comes from, the soul is described as being "pure consciousness." Writer, teacher, and Sanskrit scholar Nicolai Bachman refers to the soul, known in Sanskrit as *atman*, as the "inner light of awareness."

The soul is our reason for being incarnated in a body. Each soul has a purpose, known in Sanskrit as *dharma*. Our *dharma*, or purpose, is what we are here to learn, fulfill, or experience in this lifetime. It's not about money, power, or prestige. If it's soul-based, it has different qualities like connection, love, joy, and generosity. The biology you have is the ideal vehicle for you to fulfill your purpose.

I get asked by a lot of people, "What is my purpose?" That is an awesome question, and one that is beyond the scope of this book. It is something I believe everyone needs to figure out. Being in alignment with your purpose is health promoting. For books on the subject, check out the resources section. Stephen Cope and Simon Chokoisky have written some great books to help you find your way on the path of purpose.

From a health and healing perspective, our spirit is what inspires us. It is the reason we are here. If we are disconnected from it, this can sap our vitality and move us away from health and toward disease. Getting to know ourselves on the level of spirit (inspiration) is a powerful tool for building and maintaining health.

The Bigger Picture

In order to keep all these moving pieces working well together, Ayurveda places great emphasis on the care and management of the mind, the senses, and the soul. It is recognized that since these components coordinate and work together, it becomes important for all of these pieces to be balanced in order to attain a state of health.

They are deeply interconnected. What affects one affects the others. This is important to consider on our journey toward health. Are you taking care of all the dimensions of your being, or just one? We need to connect, care for, and heal them all to have the greatest health.

In the next section we are going to talk about the causes of disease—basically, why we get sick in the first place. You'll notice that disease can start in different places and affect different layers of your being. I believe, on some level, we already know this. ☺

CHAPTER 3

CAUSES OF DISEASE

Ayurveda describes three main causative factors in the process of disease. These are important to know because when it comes to disease, Ayurveda is all about figuring out the root cause so we can pull the weed by its roots and stop the disease from growing and spreading. It basically comes down to the things that cause our qualities to shift, and if we are unable to respond to these shifts, we get sick. It's also important to realize that illness is not limited to the body. We can have sick energy, emotions, and mind—we can have disease in any layer of our being. Where we can pay attention to the changes in the qualities, we can make choices to bring more balance into our lives.

There are many external causes of disease, like bacteria, viruses, parasites, and such. To withstand these, we must maintain strong health and immunity.

The three internal causes of disease,[39] according to Ayurveda, are:

1. Misuse of the sense organs, known as *asatmyendriyartha samyoga*[40] in Sanskrit

2. Misuse of the intellect, known as *prajnaparadha* in Sanskrit

---

39   From the *Ashtanga Samgraha, Sutrasthana 9.63.*

40   I hypothesize that this is the longest Sanskrit term in existence.

3. Change over time, known as *parinama* in Sanskrit

The internal causes of disease are the causes we have the most influence over. So we'll explore each of these in a little more depth. Before we do that, however, I want to share that for each of these detailed sections below, I will offer recommendations you can put into place to:

1. take a step in the direction of your health, and

2. influence these particular causes of disease.

It will seem like a lot of changes to make, and if you were to try to make them all it would be too much—way too much! Instead, I suggest choosing one recommendation that feels doable and commit to it daily for one month. After a month, think about whether it's supporting you or not. If it is supporting your health, keep it. If it isn't, let it go. Ayurveda is a series of scientific experiments to figure out what supports our health and what doesn't.

Once a new habit becomes part of your routine, it's time to add another one. This is a process, just like life, and it's going to take time for you to figure out the combination of diet, daily routine, and medicine of subtraction that works best for you. Remember, each step you take in the direction of your health is a step in the direction of your health! Enjoy the exploration and figuring out what works for you, one choice at a time.

Misuse of the Sense Organs

The senses are the bridge between our environment (inner and outer) and the mind. This makes their optimal functioning really important. If the sense organs aren't well maintained and/or they aren't functioning well, the information they convey to the mind will not be clear or accurate. How can you make good decisions for your health if the information you're working with is not accurate? Maintenance of the sense organs is of paramount importance. Ayurveda places a lot of time and attention on caring for the sense organs.

Misuse of the senses falls into three categories: non-use, overuse, and improper use. For each category, we can misuse any one or all of the sense organs. Ayurveda teaches us that health is about finding balance. I think of it as Goldilocks—not too much, not too little, just right. When we underuse, overuse, or misuse a sense organ, it loses its balance, becoming oversensitive or desensitized. This adjustment period then requires more energy to re-establish balance and optimal function.

Non-Use

Examples of non-use, or underuse, for each of the sense organs include:

- *Ears:* Spending too long in silence—for some people this might be an hour, for others it might be a month.

- *Skin:* Lack of loving touch.

- *Eyes:* Keeping the eyes closed for days (sleeping a lot, coma, a lot of meditation).

- *Tongue:* Fasting (no taste) or a bland diet, which in Ayurveda is a diet that does not have all six tastes[41] of sweet, sour, salty, pungent, bitter, and astringent.

---

41   More on the six tastes in the next section.

- *Nose:* Breath holding (not breathing), and bland smells and tastes (taste impacts the sense of smell).

Overuse

When the senses are overused, our nervous system (which processes the information and simultaneously governs our stress response) gets overstimulated, and then we struggle to relax and calm down. This overstimulation is a health challenge in our modern times. Here are some examples:

- *Ears:* Loud noises—music (like a rock concert), thunder, big crowds (dinner at a busy restaurant), airplanes, and the hum of technology.

- *Skin:* Extreme temperatures, bathing too frequently (multiple showers a day), too much touch (frequent massages), and the receiving line at a wedding with 200 people (touching so many people!).

- *Eyes:* Staring at a screen (TV, computer, phone, iPad, etc.) for many hours (writes the author of this book, who typed it on a laptop), flashing lights, bright objects, and not wearing sunglasses on a bright sunny day.

- *Tongue:* Eating too much or too often (too often means before the previous meal is digested) and eating only one taste (e.g., binging on sweets).

- *Nose:* Strong smells (like the perfume counter at a department store), and too much nasal oiling (*nasya*).

Improper Use

Everything your senses touch moves inside you to be processed/digested by your mind. Your response to the stimulus (whatever your sense organs take in) impacts and influences your biology. If the stimulus triggers your stress response, your entire body shifts gears to manage the stress, even if that stimulus is not real (e.g., a movie). Because your mind responds to it, so does your body. When our stress response engages, our digestion subsides, our ability to sleep is affected, and there is more hormonal wear and tear on our tissues.

Here are some examples of improper use of the sense organs:

- *Ears:* Terrifying sounds and harsh or abusive words.

- *Skin:* Physical abuse, using improper oil on your skin, suntanning, tattoos, and piercings.

- *Eyes:* Looking at things that are either very small or very large, or seeing something horrifying, frightening, scary, or anxiety-provoking (e.g., horror movies or witnessing violence or a car accident).

- *Tongue:* Food or drinks that are too hot or too cold, poor food combinations, and rotten or putrid foods.

- *Nose:* Foul, putrid, and stale smells.

In some cases we have a choice. For example, you don't have to be glued to a screen in the evenings; you can choose to unplug. Or you don't have to watch horror movies; you can turn them off.

In some cases we don't have a choice, such as witnessing an accident or hearing the sound of a busy street in the night. Some things we cannot unplug from or turn off—they are realities of life. I work with clients in professions where they see and experience horrific things (police, first responders, military, fire, and rescue). They can have "improper use of the sense organs" as an occupational hazard that is outside of their control. Caring for their sense organs and reducing their overstimulation in their off hours becomes an important way to manage occupational stress.

Ayurveda invites us to notice the ones we can influence, and to make conscious choices around these. A choice we can make is to care for our sense organs. Notice in the sections on the pillars of health how many recommendations involve the care of the sense organs.

Finding balance in the use of and health of our sense organs affects our stress response. Whether it's underuse, overuse, or improper use of the sense, at a basic level the misuse of the senses disrupts the balance of the mind. It also disrupts the clarity and purity of the information we take in from our environment, making it easier for us to "misperceive" what is going on and make poor health choices as a result. The senses are the gatekeepers of the mind. I once read: It makes sense to check ID before letting strangers into our homes. Why not use the same discretion before allowing anything into our minds through our senses? Food for thought.

Recommendations for Sense Organ Care

With the five senses being our primary gateways to awareness, proper care of the sense organs helps to clarify the messages brought in from the outside world, which allows us to make better choices for our health.

Oral Care: Mouth, Teeth, and Tongue

1. Tongue Scraping

The tongue is an important sense organ for satiation, which means feeling satisfied by your food, as it hosts the taste buds.

Preferably use a tongue scraper made of silver, copper, or stainless steel instead of plastic. Tongue scraping removes metabolic waste from the tongue and stimulates the digestive tract by awakening the taste buds.

Scrape the tongue from the root (at the back) to the tip until all the thick pasty substance is gone off the tongue. I rinse the scraper off between scrapes if there's a lot of buildup. It is helpful to rinse the mouth with water afterward.

I scrape my tongue before I brush my teeth first thing in the morning. Good to get the guck off before eating or drinking anything.

2. Teeth Brushing

This is the same tooth brushing you already know. Not all self-care practices are going to be new to you. Traditionally this was done by chewing on twigs. I like my Braun electric toothbrush. Use whatever toothbrush you have.

Clean your teeth with astringent, bitter, or pungent herbs or paste. The bitterness and astringency, as opposed to sweet and minty, help keep the gums firm and act as an oral anti-septic. Herbs traditionally used include camphor, turmeric, neem, and cloves. I am fond of the JASON Tea Tree Oil tooth-paste, which I find at the health food store.

3. Oil Holding

This technique is used when the tissues of the mouth (including teeth and gums) need more nourishment. Examples include dry mouth, tooth sensitivity, and receding gums.

Take 1 to 2 tablespoons of warm oil (sesame if you tend to be cold, or olive or coconut if you tend to be warm) and hold the liquid in your mouth for 2–15 minutes. Breathe the whole time. Then spit the oil out into the compost or garbage.

Note: Spitting oil into drains can cause clogs. Instead, I spit mine into the composter.

4. Swishing

This technique is used when there is a buildup, or stagnation, in the oral cavity. Examples of this include itching, a scratchy feeling, cankers, or halitosis.

For swishing, the recommendation is to make a *triphala infusion* to use. Triphala is an herbal formulation that is considered excellent for cleansing and clearing—it will pull the buildup out of the oral tissues.

To make the triphala infusion, take 1 teaspoon of triphala powder and soak it overnight in 1 cup of hot water (it's like making a cup of tea). The next morning, decant the infusion (this means to pour out the tea liquid, yet leave the grainy stuff in the original container).

Then use this tea for swishing. Swish for two to three minutes, then spit it out into the sink. Repeat again if you feel you need it.

5. Gargling

This can be done with warm salt water or oil.

If I use salt water, I use 1 teaspoon sea salt in 1 cup of warm (not hot) water. I stir the sea salt into the water until it dissolves. I take one mouthful at a time, lift my chin to the ceiling (no neck strain), and open my mouth and gargle for as long as I can. Then I spit the salt water into the sink and repeat until my cup of salt water is empty.

If I use oil, I take 1 tablespoon of oil, lift my chin to the ceiling (no neck strain), and open my mouth and gargle for as long as I can. Then spit the oil out into the compost or garbage.

Note: Spitting oil into drains can cause clogs. Instead, I spit mine into the composter.

Here is some extra information to clarify when you might want to use which substance:

- If I feel the beginning of a cold or a tickle in my throat, I use the sea salt water.
- If I feel dryness or scratchiness, I use the oil. The ideal oils for this are sesame, sweet almond, and olive.

Nasal Care: Nose, Nasal Passages, and Sinuses

The nose is the gateway to the head and brain. It is an important organ for breathing, and it governs the sense of smell.

1. Nasal Rinsing Using a Neti Pot and Salt Water

This technique is known as *jala neti*, in Sanskrit. *Neti* is a wonderful technique to rinse the nasal passages, clearing them in order to facilitate nasal breathing.

Neti is not recommended if you have a nosebleed or too much of the cold, heavy, thick, slimy/sticky, or liquid qualities already present in your head. I tend to be dry, so *neti* works really well for me daily. However, those who tend to be more cold, heavy, thick, slimy, and sticky might find that *neti* clears their nose for a bit, then the feeling of heavy, thick, slimy, and sticky comes back even more—remember, like increases like. No technique works for everyone all of the time. If you have too much of the cold, heavy, thick, slimy, and sticky qualities, consider a dry sauna instead of a nasal rinse.

Fill your *neti* pot with clean warm water and sea salt. The sea salt measurement is about ½–1 teaspoon sea salt for each cup of water. The idea is to adjust the water to the salinity (or saltiness) of your own tears. If you ever try it without salt, it will create a burning sensation in your nose. Ironically, the same thing will happen if there's too much salt. Like Goldilocks, we're looking for a balanced place of "just right."

Once the pot and salt water are set up, allow the water to flow through the nasal passages with gravity. It is not recommended to sniff the water up into the nose or to use any forceful means that can damage sensitive nasal tissues. You can add a bit of baking soda (half the amount of the salt) to the mix if your nasal tissues are very dry or sensitive.

I have a family member who used to get sinus infections every winter—sometimes up to five each winter. Each sinus infection led to a course of antibiotics. And thank goodness for the antibiotics to fight the infection; however, we all know that taking a lot of antibiotics isn't good for us. I taught this person to *neti*, and their sinus infections went down from every winter to maybe one infection every other winter. It's an effective technique, for sure. And it's interesting because the *neti* water doesn't actually go into your sinuses. What happens is that the clearing of the nostrils and nasal passages keeps "stuff" from building up and blocking the sinuses. It allows mucous and accumulation to flow out of the sinuses into the nasal passages for elimination, which means it supports the proper flow through these channels.

Note: For this recommendation, **I strongly recommend getting instruction from someone with experience using a *neti* pot.** The way you position your head and body makes a difference in terms of getting the water to flow through the proper channels in your head—in one nostril and out the other, instead of in one nostril and down the throat.

2. Oil Your Nostrils

This oiling of the nose is known as *nasya* in Sanskrit. This practice is a follow-up to the nasal rinsing. Once your nostrils are clear and clean, oil the nostrils to nourish and strengthen the mucous membranes of the nose. The nose is the entry point of air, which often has all sorts of stuff in it, including debris, pollution, and bacteria/viruses. Strong nasal tissue keeps all that stuff from getting into your bloodstream—it's one of our lines of defense against infection and sickness. One to two drops into each nostril does the trick. Sometimes I put a bit of oil onto my pinky fingertips and rub them gently along the inside of each nostril. You can use sesame, *ghee*, or sweet almond oil. In this case, a little bit goes a long way.

Eye Care

1. Eye Rinse

The eyes are our most delicate sense organ. The eyes may be cleansed daily by rinsing with fresh clean water. I cup my hands under the tap and collect cool water, then I bring it up to my eyes and splash the water on my face and blink my eyes to gently let the water in.

I am blessed to live where the tap water is potable. If you don't have potable tap water, boil the water (rolling boil) for three to five minutes, let it cool to room temperature, then use it as instructed above. Otherwise, you can purchase distilled water.

2. Rose Water

A way to cool down and soothe the eyes when the eyes are hot and strained is to use a rose water dilution. I find this works really well after hours at the computer, or when my eyes feel tired after a day in the sun. This practice is not meant to be a daily practice, as the rose water dilution can be drying to the eyes if done too often. It is practiced as needed, and as long as you don't already have dry eyes (meaning, don't do this if you have dry eyes already).

It's important that we are really clear about what rose water is: The rose water I am talking about is a steam distillation using organic rose petals. To make the rose water for your eyes, in a spray bottle mix 1 part rose water distillation to 3–4 parts regular water. It's important to dilute the rose water so the eyes don't get dried out.

For the technique, mist the diluted rose water into the space in front of your face, as though you were spraying your whole face, and blink to allow some of the rose water dilution into your eyes. While you're doing this, take a deep breath to "smell the roses." You could also use an eye cup and blink the rose water into your eyes, one eye at a time, and using a fresh amount of rose water for each eye.

Note: What rose water is NOT is water with rose essential oil in it. DO NOT put essential oils in your eyes. Also, do not bring the pump right up to your eye like you were flushing it after getting debris in it. Both of these things could damage your eyes.

3. Triphala Infusion

If your eyes get a thick sticky goopeyness, rinse the eyes using a *triphala infusion*. Triphala is an herbal formulation that is considered excellent for cleansing and clearing—it will pull the thick sticky stuff out of the eyes.

To make the triphala infusion, take 1 teaspoon of triphala powder and soak it overnight in 1 cup of hot water (it's like making a cup of tea). The next morning, decant the infusion (this means to pour out the tea liquid, yet leave the grainy stuff in the original container) through a coffee filter to get the liquid without the grit. Then use an eye cup to rinse out each eye, one at a time. Use new triphala infusion for each eye, meaning if you use 2 tablespoons for the right eye, then after rinsing the right eye, dump it down the sink and take a new 2 tablespoons to rinse the left eye.

This technique is not done daily but as needed. It is not recommended more than once per week.

4. Ghee

If your eyes get dry, high-quality clear *ghee* (clarified butter) can be applied on the inside upper and lower eyelids (where eyeliner goes) before sleep.

Ears

1. Oil Your Ears

Dip the tip of your little finger into warm oil (whatever you use for your nostrils or skin works), then insert the little finger into the ear and gently rotate it around the aperture. A few drops of oil can be inserted directly into the ear canal as well. This helps to reduce ear canal dryness and ringing in the ears.

Note: Caution must be taken if you wear hearing aids, as the oil can wreck the hearing aid. If you have a hearing impairment and want to try this technique, perhaps do it before bed once you've taken your hearing aids out for the night. And remember to check with your MD first!

Skin

1. Dry Brushing

This is done with a raw silk glove before taking a shower or bath. The entire body benefits from this technique. Some sources recommend daily, others weekly, and others seasonally (this is a great practice for the spring season). This is a helpful practice if your lymphatic and circulatory systems tend to be sluggish (if you have stagnation), or if your skin gets itchy. Be careful with dry or aging skin, as well as with the face and genital regions. If you have super dry skin, it's best to skip this.

For dry brushing, begin at your feet and work your way up the body. Use long strokes (back and forth) across the long bones, and circular motions (round and round) at the joints, abdomen, low back, and breasts.

Note: Remember to wash your raw silk gloves regularly and hang them dry.

2. Self-Oil Massage

Self-oil massage, called *abhyanga* in Sanskrit, is a staple practice in the world of Ayurveda. In the fall and winter use sesame or sweet almond oil, in the spring use sunflower oil, and in the summer use coconut.

REMEMBER: DO NOT apply any substance that you are allergic or sensitive to! Be mindful that what goes on the skin is digested through the skin and moves right into the bloodstream.

Oil massage nourishes, strengthens, and protects the seven layers of the skin. It improves immunity by stimulating the lymphatic, circulatory, and eliminatory systems. It is also soothing for the nervous system as it harmonizes the flow of *prana* (vital energy). This is a great technique if your nerves need settling, if you feel cold often, or if your skin is dry and rough. This is not recommended if your skin is already oily or you feel heavy and congested.

When massaging, use circular motions at the joints, abdomen, low back, and breasts, and long strokes (up and down) over the long bones and side torso. You don't need to do a lot of strokes; you only have to get the oil on your skin, then let the oil do the work of nourishing you.

Apply the oil before showering, then wait 5–15 minutes before going into the shower or tub so the oil absorbs into your skin. Maybe apply the oil, then brush your teeth, or take five minutes to breathe and meditate. Once in the shower/tub, rinse your body first, allowing the pores to open and the oil to go deep into the tissues. Then soap off any excess oil, as well as the hair-covered portions of your body (pits and bits—armpits and groin area). Once done, pat dry.

Additional Tips for Self-Oiling:

- If you are purchasing big containers of oil, keep the main jar in the refrigerator (so it lasts longer, as "good" oils eventually spoil) and keep a small bottle or jar in the bathroom for easy access.

- To warm your oil, put the sealed bottle of oil in a cup of hot water. I use a plastic container to hold the water because my oil jars are glass and I broke one once when the glass of my oil jar hit the glass container holding the hot water. It was messy. My friend Veronica fills a mini slow cooker with water and lets the oil jar sit in the heated water to warm up. It works really well.

- Use oil appropriate for your skin, the season, or any

imbalance you are working with. The head, scalp, and face might need different oil than the body.

- There are some days I do not have time for a full-body self-oil massage. On those days I massage my feet and low back for grounding, and my arms because they get a lot of use and touch a lot of things. The classical texts recommend oiling the head, ears, and feet.

- If you have oil on your head (which likely also means in your hair), then avoid going outside in the winter (cold) and on a windy day. If it's winter or windy season, then do the head oiling in the evening before bed and wash the oil out and dry your hair before going outside.

- When you are doing self-massage, remember to do it with an attitude of self-love—you'll get so much more out of it! Acting with love releases oxytocin, a love hormone that promotes tissue regeneration and rejuvenation. You can do this technique as a "forced march," but you won't get as much benefit from it.

3. Daily Shower or Bath

After the sense organs have been cleansed, bathing is the single most important practice for maintaining cleanliness and longevity. Showers and baths are invigorating, cleansing, and soothing to the body-mind, which becomes pliable and refreshed. Water is great to wash away dirt and negative energies.

4. Daily Sweating

One of the best things for the skin is sweating. Sweating opens the pores and allows toxins and wastes to move through these channels for elimination. It is recommended that you sweat a little bit daily to keep the skin healthy.

Sweating can happen from the inside or the outside—and both work. An example of sweating from the inside is exercise, where you warm the body up enough that sweating happens. An example of sweating from the outside includes saunas, steam rooms, or hot showers.

Do your best to sweat a little bit every day, and you'll notice a difference in the health of your skin.

In terms of how sweating fits in with the skin care regimen, it depends on how you are sweating. If you choose to sweat from exercise, then the recommended order is exercise, oil massage, and then shower. If you choose to sweat through the sauna, then the recommended order is oil massage, sauna (with the oil on your skin—the sauna will increase the absorption of the oil through the opening of the pores), then bath.

Sense Care Conclusion

Given that our sense organs are the gateway between everything and our brains, taking care of our senses so we can receive accurate information about our environment is very important. Sense organ care is a great place to start taking a step in the direction of your health. Consider which of your sense organs would benefit from support and start there. Or choose something that feels doable and start doing it.

Misuse of the Intellect

This one is fascinating. My favourite translation of the Sanskrit for this cause of disease is "intellectual blasphemy." Doesn't that sound intriguingly dramatic? And even more interesting is that everyone I know—including me!—does this in some way, shape, or form.

Misuse of the Intellect basically means one of two things (or both of them):

1. Doing something you know is not good for you
2. Not doing something you know is good for you

The first aspect of misuse of the mind is where you know something is not good for you, and you do it anyway. An example is sitting in front of the TV and eating an entire bag of chips while watching Netflix, or smoking cigarettes. No human being needs to eat an entire bag of chips (unless you were stranded on a desert island and were starving, which is not a common experience in our modern day). This puts too much food in your belly, taxes your digestive fire, and clogs your channels (more on this when we talk about the first pillar of health), which is not going to support your health. And there is no science out there that says smoking has any benefit whatsoever. If anything, we know it causes many diseases (from COPD to cancer), and yet we continue to smoke cigarettes.

Just so we're clear, I smoked for ten years (and not during the time when we didn't know smoking was hazardous!) and have absolutely eaten a bag of chips while binging on Netflix. I'm not saying any of this to be righteous; I'm being factual and honest because loving honesty is important and necessary for health. I am grateful for the teachers who pointed out to me where I was choosing my own suffering instead of choosing health and happiness. That's the whole point of this book.

There are things we know take away from our health, and we do them anyway. We often create our own suffering. Heck, sometimes we even know we're going to suffer as a result of making a choice! I have a great example of this. I was asked once for an Ayurvedic remedy to cure a hangover for a New Year's Day social media post. My response was: Don't get drunk on New Year's Eve. Ayurveda isn't magic—it is common sense. If you don't want the hangover, don't get drunk. Straight line, easy-peasy. However, how many people choose to drink in excess, despite knowing that they will be sick the next day? This is intellectual blasphemy.

We also misuse our mind when we know something is good for us but choose not to do it. An example of this is not exercising, not getting enough sleep, or not eating enough veggies. We know all these things are health promoting—they are good for us—and yet we make excuses (we misuse the power of our minds) to not do these health-promoting practices. I see, and also do, this one all the time.

There are multiple categories of misuse of the intellect. The first is verbal impropriety, things like lying or speaking abusive words. The second is mental impropriety, which is where we do things that make the mind dull or agitated instead of balanced. The third is physical impropriety, which includes overwork, the suppression of natural urges, and improper eating.

This means there are three levels where we can misuse the

intellect, but really it all comes down to knowing something's good for you and not doing it, or knowing something's bad for you and doing it anyway.

Recommendations for Your Mind

1. Meditation

Meditation techniques are designed to help us self-observe: to notice when our mind is calm, agitated, or dull. Having this self-awareness helps us to know if the information we're working with is accurate or not. You can work with any form of meditation that resonates with you, from Yoga Nidra to Loving Kindness to Mindfulness to Open Palm. A regular meditation practice has been shown to reduce stress.

One of the simplest meditation techniques is breath awareness meditation. Find a comfortable seat (if you aren't comfortable, you'll be constantly distracted by the discomfort) and settle in. Soften your gaze. If it feels safe, close your eyes. Let your body relax and focus on the natural flow of your breath. Natural breath means that you watch your breath as it is; no need to change it by making it longer or slowing it down, simply notice your breath. Then pay attention, as full of attention as you can, to your breathing. Notice the in-breaths (known as inhalations) and the out-breaths (known as exhalations). Notice if your breath makes sound or is quiet—listen to your breath. Notice where in your body the breath creates movement—feel your breath.

Your mind is going to want to do other things, like make grocery lists and explore deep contemplations about what's happening in the next season of *Brooklyn Nine-Nine*. When you notice your mind has wandered in this way, simply and patiently bring your focus back to watching your breath.

This teaches us to point our mind in one place and sustain that focus amidst the distractions of life. If you want to do anything, you have to be able to focus on it. Meditation can help you with this. A mind that can focus can also choose to focus on things that bring us balance.

If you're new to meditation, I highly recommend finding a good teacher to guide you. It made all the difference in the world for me, as a student of meditation, to have a good teacher to help me.

2. Time in Nature

Nature calms and settles the mind and senses. Another way of saying this is nature is *sattvic*, and like increases like. This could be going for a walk outside, taking a hike at the conservation area, or working in your very own garden. Time spent in nature also reduces stress.

3. Positive Affirmations or Mantra

Affirmations are statements of intention—what we want to experience or the trajectory we want to move in. *Mantras* are ancient sacred sound vibrations that cultivate *sattvic* energies. They use repetition to pattern the mind; we could say they train the mind to flow in a particular way. These tools are useful to help us establish new patterns of thought and behaviour, to create new habits.

Mind Care Conclusion

Finding a way to balance the mind makes a huge difference in our overall health. When the mind finds balance, it's very straightforward for the rest of our layers of being to find balance too. It took me a few years to figure it out; however, I do at least one thing every day to care for my mind, and it is a game changer. Consider which of the three recommendations above you're willing to try to care for your mind.

Change over Time

There are natural, and fairly predictable, fluctuations that happen within each of us. We have shifts in our qualities over the course of the day, month, year (think seasons), and life-time (think of childhood, middle age, the golden years). As our qualities change with these natural environmental and life shifts, they have the significant potential to throw our systems out of balance.

Have you ever noticed that …

… people tend to get sick during the change in season?

… children tend to be more resilient (health wise) than the elderly?

… women have different levels of stability at different times of the month based on their menstrual cycle?

This concept of change over time is not something we can control—far from it. It's something that happens to everyone, no matter what. According to Ayurveda, this is one of the two strongest influences on our health (for those who are wondering, the other is food).

Now, we may not be able to control the weather, how old we are, or what time of day it is, yet we can learn how to respond to these shifts in a way that helps us stay more balanced. That way, we don't get far enough out of balance for disease to take hold.

Seasons

The atmospheric changes that are created with the change in season affect all living things, which includes us, as we are part of nature. Since the seasons are a force of great substance, Ayurveda has always recommended we align ourselves with the seasons, with the rhythms of nature. Seasons are different in different parts of the world, and so it is helpful to look at the qualities of the seasons, in order to determine which qualities we need to balance. It often comes down to recognizing the qualities and responding to this increase by applying the opposite quality.

Ayurveda offers suggestions to maximize the positive benefits of these changes, as well as minimize any negative implications. Lack of compensation for the changes in season (or time of life) can result in imbalance, which can lead to illness and disease. It is not always possible to completely neutralize the adverse effects of environmental factors; however, simple adjustments definitely help. This is known as *seasonal regimen*.

Northern Solstice—Spring and Summer Seasons

During this time, both the sun and wind become strong, and we see an *increase in the hot and dry qualities*. This removes the cooling qualities from the earth. The same effect occurs with all living beings and plants. The increase in heat reduces strength and lowers appetite. Pathogens are in abundance. The grains and vegetables that grow are predominantly pungent, bitter, and astringent in taste (lightening/cleansing tastes). These tastes protect the body from overgrowth (of tissues, pathogens, and microbes) through natural detoxification.

Southern Solstice—Fall and Winter Seasons

During this time, the earth's orbit around the sun takes the earth far away from the sun. This means that the moon is more powerful, and the earth *cools* down by the effects of clouds, rain, snow, and cold wind. Resistance to disease is naturally stronger at this time, and so health is maintained.

The harvests for the fall and winter seasons contain predominantly sweet, salty, and sour tastes, which have qualities that build tissues and nourish the body.

In terms of seasonal changes, Ayurveda describes three stages of change in the qualities:

1. Accumulation, known as *sanchaya* in Sanskrit: this is the stage where a quality starts to increase or build.

2. Aggravation, known as *prakopa* in Sanskrit: this is the stage where the buildup of a quality starts to move you out of balance.

3. Alleviation, known as *prashama* in Sanskrit: this is the stage where an opposite quality naturally increases, balancing out the imbalance in a natural way.

Qualities increase and are provoked during the seasonal changes. The last week of the outgoing season and the first week of the incoming season, totalling 15 days, are the most challenging to balance. During this junction, the previous season's regimen gradually declines as we shift into the regimen for the upcoming season.

In North America (which is where this author is from), this occurs from fall to winter, winter to spring, spring to summer, and summer to fall. Other geographic areas have their own seasons and seasonal transitions. You'll have to explore what seasons you have, and what the effects are on the increase and decrease of qualities. The classical Ayurvedic text, written in India, describes the six seasons common to the Indian climate. It has been interesting to see how these ancient teachings are being adapted to modern day, and to other climates and environments.

The change in seasons is a common time for illness to take hold. It is important to take time to check in with yourself, to center, and to adjust as you need to for these changes. A client once asked me, "What happens if the weather is always the same where I live?" (she lived in a tropical and consistent climate), and I replied, "Then you don't have to worry about adjusting your routine for the seasonal change. However, there is a higher risk that certain qualities will build, so you'll need to make sure you eat and live in alignment with your environment." For her that meant eating cooling foods (to balance the hot climate), not overworking (to keep from overheating), and ensuring ample hydration (to balance the dryness and moisture loss from a climate that has the body constantly sweating).

Spring Transition

Spring is a season of growth and renewal (birth) in the annual cycle. It is connected to *kapha dosha* (due to an increase in the *kapha* qualities of heavy, slow/dull, cold, oily, smooth, soft, stable, obvious, and cloudy/sticky/slimy), childhood in the cycle of life, and the postmenstrual growth phase in the lunar cycle.

1. *Accumulation:* The cool quality begins to accumulate throughout the fall and even more with the onset of winter as the planet moves further from the sun and the days get shorter. The heavy quality also accumulates with the heavy and dense foods eaten in the winter.

2. *Aggravation:* Heavy, dense, thick, and slimy qualities aggravate in the spring, as the heat liquefies the accumulation, turning it into mucous. You might notice congestion, some swelling of your hands and feet, and a sense of heaviness in your body. The early actions to reduce aggravation include hot herbal steam bath, herbal paste application (known as *urdvartana*), and oiling your nostrils (known as *nasya*).

3. *Alleviation:* The mucous (heavy, dense, thick, slimy, sticky qualities) reduction occurs naturally in the summer with its light, dry, and hot qualities.

Over the course of winter, the qualities of springtime have

been building. When spring arrives, with its moist, heavy, cloudy, soft, and cool qualities, any accumulation of these in the body aggravates and we end up with congestion, swelling, foggy minds, sluggish digestion, and excess weight. We might also feel lonely, worried, sad, or depressed.

Ayurveda offers a myriad of ways to create balance during the spring season. We can do this through diet and lifestyle choices. I will go into these in more detail in the third pillar of health when we cover the daily routine.

Summer Transition

In the summer, the earth is closest to the sun it's going to get! Summer is a season of work (heat) and cultivation (reap what you sowed) in the annual cycle. It is related to *pitta dosha* (due to an increase in the *pitta* qualities of hot, sharp, penetrating, light, slightly oily, liquid, spreading, and flesh smelling) and represents adulthood in the cycle of life, and the premenstrual phase in the lunar cycle.

1. *Accumulation:* The hot and liquid qualities begin to accumulate from spring to summer due to the change from cool and dry to hot and damp.

2. *Aggravation:* As the summer gets hotter, the hot and liquid qualities increase to the point of aggravation. You might notice an increase in liquid bowel movements and heat in the body (a lot of sweating, hot flashes, and irritability). The early actions to reduce aggravation include oiling with cooling or neutral oil (like coconut, sunflower, or *ghee*), herbal steam baths, and head oiling (known as *shirodhara*) with cooling herbs.

3. *Alleviation:* The qualities reduce naturally in the fall as the temperatures cool down and the environment becomes drier in nature.

Over the course of spring, the qualities of summer build, specifically heat and moisture. Therefore, when summer arrives, with its hot, sharp, light, and moist qualities, any accumulation of heat in the body aggravates, and we end up with rashes, acne (all sorts of skin stuff), acidity, inflammation, and hyper-digestion. We might also feel irritated, angry, frustrated, critical, and dissatisfied.

Fall Transition

Fall is the season of unwinding and settling into the annual cycle. It is connected to *vata dosha* (due to an increase in the *vata* qualities of cold, light, dry, rough, mobile, subtle, and clear) and represents the golden years in the cycle of life, and the menstrual phase in the lunar cycle.

1. *Accumulation:* In the late summer, the digestive fire is weaker and the body's water levels are low due to perspiration. The dry and light qualities of the summer are dominant in nature (this includes you!) and food.

2. *Aggravation:* As the cold and dry qualities become dominant, they aggravate in the late fall and early winter. You might notice an increase in dryness (skin, tongue, hair, and eyes), as well as an increase in the cold quality (hands, fingers, feet, and catching a cold). The early actions to reduce aggravation include self-oil massage and sweat therapy, because both are warming and oily.

3. *Alleviation:* There is a natural reduction of the qualities that occur in the spring as the humidity and heat increase in the environment. Depending on the qualities present in the winter, we may get some alleviation in winter; however, sometimes we have to wait until spring. You can read more about that in the section below on winter.

The heat of summer dries out the environment, which increases the dry quality. When fall arrives, the cold and mobile qualities are increased, and this combination of cold, mobile, and dry aggravates our systems. You might notice dryness in the skin, hair, mouth, and throat, more stiffness in your body, and pain showing back up when you thought it had gone away. Our digestion can become variable—one minute we are starving, and then we forget to eat the next meal because there was no hunger. We might also feel spacey, overwhelmed, anxious, or fearful.

Winter Transition

Winter is the season of hibernation in the annual cycle. It represents death in the cycle of life and menopause as its associated menstrual phase.

Winter in North America is interesting when observed through this lens. The cold quality continues to increase, accumulate, and aggravate; yet the accompanying qualities differ from winter to winter. Some winters are more cold and dry (like the fall season), while others are cold and moist with wet snow or heavy snow (like the spring season), and a third option is swinging between a fall-like winter and a spring-like winter.

When the winters are cold and dry, we continue to follow the regimen prescribed for fall. If the winter is cold and moist, then we follow the regimen prescribed for spring. Even more interesting is that as I write this, the winter that just passed (2017–2018) was both. One day it was –32 degrees Celsius with cold, dry, and clear skies and a bright sun (yet still –32°C!). The next day it was –6°C with wet snow. The pendulum kept swinging back and forth, from extreme to extreme. As a result, a lot of people were sick, and they stayed sick longer. Their systems were unable to stabilize and find balance amidst all the seasonal changes.

Seasonal Routine Conclusion

What we choose in terms of our diet, daily routine, and self-care practices can profoundly influence the qualities we embody and either support their balance or imbalance. As we interact with the world, the qualities shift and change and can go out of balance, creating disease. By aligning with the rhythms of nature, starting with recognizing what we need from season to season, we are better able to keep our qualities and ourselves in balance. Maintaining health (prevention) is easier than treating disease.

Section Conclusion

I suspect it's becoming clearer that, although there are many things in the world we have no control over, there are a lot of things that we can do to bring some balance into our lives through awareness and conscious action. As we move into the next section, we'll talk about the power of choice, and how, now that we understand the three internal causes of disease, we have a choice in how we want to work with that information.

CHAPTER 4

POWER OF CHOICE

Ayurveda guides us to the realization that our health is created by our daily choices. It is rarely one big thing, although every once in a while, it is. For the most part, health is about choosing the healthy option, when we can figure out what that is.

Every step you take in the direction of your health is a step in the direction of your health. I know it sounds obvious and simplistic, yet it is still 100% accurate! The more of these steps we take, the healthier we become. It comes down to choosing health.

The main obstacles I see in my clients, and that I encounter in myself, are our likes and dislikes, which I call "preferences." Sometimes the healthy choice means letting go of something I think I like, or choosing something that I dislike. The interesting thing about our preferences is that they change over time. If this is one of your challenges, I invite you to think about why you like the things you like, and why you dislike the things you dislike. I also invite you to think about changing your mind. What would happen if you chose to like the things that support your health simply because they support your health? What if you chose to dislike the things that take away from your health because they take away from your health? Would that make things easier on you? Would this help you choose your health? Over the years of working toward health, I have learned to love the things that support my health. I know what they are and when to use them.

Given all the pieces to the puzzle—the multifaceted nature of our being and the causes of disease—it can be challenging to see the road we need to travel. This is where the three pillars of health come in. Ayurveda gives us a map to help us make healthy choices. The bulk of the book is about these three pillars and how to strengthen them.

In the end, it comes down to you. What will you choose? You can choose health or not choose health. The power is in your choices, day to day, moment to moment. I know you can do this because I've done it. I am not special, gifted, or talented in the realms of health. If you read the introduction, you know I've had my fair share of health disasters. What I learned is that my health is a result of the choices I make. When I owned that and started to choose my health, I got healthier. When I step off the trail and don't choose my health, I don't get healthier. It is that simple.

This proactive self-care is really important. No one will care as much about your health and well-being as you do—and, frankly, so it should be! A lot of people think that by investing time in their self-care they are being selfish. I argue the opposite actually. If you spend some time every day taking care of yourself, then you can show up and give fully of yourself in your life—whether that be for family, at work, or at play. If you don't take care of yourself and you get sick, then others have to take care of you. I believe investing in our self-care is being self-invested, not selfish.

Consider self-care as preventive medicine. It's about setting yourself up so that you are less likely to get sick, because you are choosing your health every day. And this is the essence of the Ayurvedic teachings. Ayurveda is a health care system designed to **maintain the health of the healthy person** first and foremost. This is where Ayurveda rocks! And for any of you who, like me, have been really sick before, it is a full-time job to get your health back when you lose it. The simpler choice is to maintain the health you have and build it up one step at a time.

Each day I ask myself one question, "What will I choose to do for my health today?"

And so I ask you: *"What will you choose to do for your health today?"*

SECTION II:

PILLAR 1

NOURISHMENT

Let food be thy medicine and medicine be thy food.

—Hippocrates

Introduction to Pillar 1

Ayurveda's first pillar of health is nourishment, called *ahara* in Sanskrit. This is a huge and multidimensional topic. Get ready—we're going for a ride!

From the Ayurvedic view, nourishment includes everything we take into the body-mind: food, water, breath, information, experiences, energy, emotions, thoughts, company, and all the sensory impressions. This means that nourishment isn't only about what you take into your body in terms of food, it's about everything you take into your body-mind-spirit. Remember, from the Ayurvedic perspective you are more than just a body. You are a body, energy, emotions, mind, bliss, and spirit all in one package!

Why is nourishment important?

The nourishment we take in becomes us! What we ingest, after being digested, literally gets transformed into our actual tissues. If we want a strong and healthy body, we need to nourish our tissues.

Vagbhata, author of one of Ayurveda's authoritative texts, says:

> Authorities say that food and drink partaken in a proper manner only, are helpful for satisfying the senses and bestowing long life. On it, depends the valour, growth, nourishment, intelligence, and health of the person. It is

fuel for the internal fire and this fire is the chief support of the body.[42]

If we are not well nourished, our tissues lose their strength, stability, and resilience. When our tissues deplete or weaken (sometimes we can end up with a lot of tissue, but not good-quality tissue), we get sick, tired, lethargic, achy, and out of balance. Our tissues are what make up our channels, so if the tissues are not healthy, our channels aren't healthy, and we aren't healthy. In order for us to produce good-quality tissues, we need good-quality nourishment.

What we take in affects the body, our senses (moods and reactions), the balance of our mind (our thoughts and beliefs), and our ability to stay connected to our spirit. This means that nourishment can support or deplete our body (tissues), senses, energy, mood, mind, and heart too.

How do I know if something is nourishing for me?

Ayurveda believes that every substance in the world has the potential to be medicine or poison. From broccoli to your iPhone to the people you spend time with—each has the potential to support your health or deplete it. How do we know if something is healing or toxic for us? Ayurveda tells us that if you can digest it, it nourishes you, and if you cannot, it causes disease. This applies to food AND energies, emotions, thoughts, beliefs, and experiences. We are, after all, more than our bodies.

I find it very useful to ask myself, "Is this nourishing or toxic?" I also find it helpful to notice how I feel after consuming

---

42   From the *Ashtanga Samgraha, Sutrasthana 10.2.*

something. If it's nourishing, you will feel vibrant, alive, enthusiastic, and light. If it isn't, it's likely that you'll feel heavy, dense, sluggish, and ready for a nap. Anything that depletes your system is not nourishing, even if we think it is (prime example of misuse of the mind!).

The truth is, for a lot of things, it depends. In my experience, there are additional pieces to this part of the puzzle: quality, quantity, and context.

Quality

The first consideration is the quality of what you are consuming. We know that there are different qualities of nourishment available to us. There is a difference between fresh local fruits and vegetables and freeze-dried food packaged in a wrapper. The same holds true with the company we keep. There is a difference between someone who honours who you are and treats you with kindness and respect, and someone who does not. The same is true of media and entertainment—this is everything from TV and movies to newspapers, plays, music, concerts, books, webinars … you name it! Some entertainment uplifts, inspires, and connects us to the world around us, while others are full of terrifying, enraging, anxiety-provoking content that disconnects us from each other.

Ayurveda invites us to choose quality nourishment in terms of our food, our experiences, and the company we keep.

Quantity

Another consideration is the quantity we are consuming. It is absolutely possible to consume something high quality that becomes indigestible at high quantities. I think about this as a dosage issue. Consider these examples.

If you have a headache and you take one aspirin for it, and your headache goes away: Good dosage = Medicine. If you take the whole bottle of aspirin, you will overdose and end up in the hospital: Incorrect dosage = Poison. It's the same substance, but the difference is the quantity consumed: the dose.

This can apply to food too! My favourite example is chocolate (chocolate is my favourite food in the whole world!). If I eat a piece of organic natural dark chocolate, not only is it yummy for my taste buds, but it is also digestible and yummy for my body and my mind. However, if I eat three family-size chocolate bars (even if they are still organic, refined sugar–free, and fair-trade dark chocolate), there is a point where I can no longer digest the amount, or dosage, of the food that I am taking in. It stops being yummy to my system and starts being yucky and toxic.

Dr. John Douillard told our class that the average American eats 100% more than they actually need for their health and survival. There can be "too much of a good thing."

Context

When I talk about *context*, I'm referring to a few things.

First, context refers to *each individual person*. Ayurveda is very clear in its belief that there is no *one size fits all* for health. Every person is unique, and that means every person will need their own unique combination of the three pillars of health in order to find health, balance, and well-being. This is why in an Ayurvedic practice, we see clients one-on-one because everyone is different and requires their own unique regimen.[43]

Back to context as individuality. Here we want to understand that it is not just about the substance being consumed. I've noticed that every year there is a new "superfood" promoted: from quinoa to kale to garlic to turmeric. I'm glad we are developing awareness around how food can nourish us, but it is a mistake to think that one food will be equally nourishing for everyone. I know someone who is allergic to turmeric. Should she still eat turmeric because it's a superfood? Absolutely not! For some people, turmeric is very healing, yet for her it's poisonous and she needs to stay away from it in order to be healthy. We cannot assume that what works for us will work for someone else, or that what works for someone else will work for us. We're all different, and we need different things to maintain our health.

Context also refers to the *situation the person is in*. Whether you are happy, sad, tired, angry, stressed, relaxed, working too hard, or on holiday—all these contextual pieces influence your ability to digest something.

One example of this is grief. In my experience, grief is "digestive overload." When I'm in it, it doesn't matter what I take in, it is not nourishing me because I am not able to digest much during those times.

Another example is stressed versus relaxed. This one is wired

---

43   I acknowledge that saying this and then writing a book of general trends and recommendations is ironic. The more you get to know me, the more you'll see how much I love irony.

right into our biology. Our nervous system governs a lot of what is going on for us. I think of it as the manager of our body-mind. It has two main modes: "active/fight or flight" and "rest and digest." If I am working really hard, always on the go, and not sleeping, will I be able to digest? Probably not, because I'm not getting into "rest and digest" mode. If I make time to sit and eat, to unwind from my busy day, and I am able to sleep, now will I be able to digest? There is a good chance I will because I am able to get into "rest and digest" mode.

Context can also refer to *which layer of being is getting nourished*. I've learned over the years that what nourishes one layer of my being might not nourish another. Life isn't always simple, and this is no different. Sometimes the answer is simple, like protein builds muscle tissue. Sometimes the answer isn't, like should I stay up until 3 a.m. and eat at the midnight poutine bar the night of my brother's wedding? That's more complicated. And even if my body paid the price for eating midnight poutine and staying up until 3 a.m., my heart would not have missed being at my brother's wedding for the world!

Quality, quantity, and context for nourishment matters, and yet they are all dependent on our ability to digest what we take in. This is why digestion is a central concept in Ayurveda. Most Ayurvedic recommendations are to support and maintain strong digestion so that what we take in can actually nourish us. Let's dive deeper into a key piece of the puzzle, something Ayurveda calls *agni*, our digestive potential.

CHAPTER 5

IMPORTANCE OF DIGESTION

*A*gni is the Sanskrit word that refers to our digestive potential, our biological fire, the heat energy that governs our
metabolism. Our digestive potential is responsible for digesting our food, sensory impressions, experiences, emotions,
and ideas. Ayurveda believes that our ability to take in and
process, to digest and integrate everything that happens in
our life, comes down to the capacity and the strength of our
agni.

In Ayurveda the fire element represents the strength of our
digestive potential and is also connected to the brilliance
of our mind, our intelligence. One aspect of *agni* is the fire
in the belly that digests our food. Another aspect of *agni* is
the fire of the mind that digests our emotions, thoughts, and
experiences. What I find fascinating about this is how many
people "know" something "in their gut." This shows us the
connection between the fire of the mind and the fire of the
belly. Ayurveda explains that fire is fire. It's all the same fire;
it is simply performing different functions.

The stronger our fire, digestive or otherwise, the stronger our
inner knowing and our ability to get the answers we need from
within. In yoga, we refer to this as our "inner teacher," and
it is our innate intelligence. This is important because what
works for someone else might not work for you, because you
are unique. One of the things Ayurveda is trying to help us

with is finding the answers for our own health and well-being within ourselves. In order to do this, we have to support and strengthen *agni*.

When our *agni* becomes diminished, this impairs our ability to understand, as well as our ability to sink into our own self and access information and answers.

What Does *Agni* Do?

As we put things into our bodies, our digestive potential has a variety of functions.

First is awareness and intelligence. *Agni* has to figure out what we've ingested, so it knows how to break it down and how to digest it. This matters because if we can't break down the food we take in, our body can't get nourishment from it, which means our tissues weaken and deplete. I also think this comes into play with knowing what to eat and when to eat it.

Second is discernment. After *agni* breaks things down into smaller pieces, it has to figure out which pieces to keep (nourishment) and which pieces to get rid of (elimination of wastes). This is important because if the body mixes these things up, we lose our nourishment and hold onto toxic materials. This need for discernment happens outside of our stomach too. Knowing what we need in our life in order to nourish ourselves, and what we need to let go of and move on from, is relevant to our health.

Third is transformation. *Agni* takes the nourishment and changes it into energy and tissues that build the body-mind. If this isn't happening, we get tired and depleted. I believe humans are wired for growth and evolution—for transformation. If we're not growing in some way, we get tired and depleted.

Charaka, one of Ayurveda's source authors, describes *agni* in this way:

> Agni is the "raison d'etre" of life, complexion, strength, health, enthusiasm, plumpness (energy), *ojas* (immunity), *tejas* (radiance), and *prana* (the vital breath). Extinction of this *agni* leads to death; its proper maintenance helps a person to live a long life, and its impairment gives rise to diseases. Therefore *agni* is considered to be the root or the most important sustaining factor of living beings.[44]

> Food provides nourishment to the tissues and *ojas* (vital essence of immunity), strength, complexion, but in effect it is the *agni* that plays a vital role in this connection because tissue elements cannot originate from undigested food particles.[45]

Charaka clearly explains how important *agni* is, not only for you to digest your food, but in order for you to have immunity, energy, and health.

---

44   From the *Charaka Samhita, Chikitsasthana 15.3–4.*

45   From the *Charaka Samhita, Chikitsasthana 15.5.*

How Do I Know If My *Agni* Is Healthy?

Ayurveda teaches that there are four kinds of *agni*:[46]

1. Balanced
2. Sharp
3. Slow
4. Variable

We are going to monitor our digestive potential using the following tools: hunger, what is happening in our digestive tract, and bowel movements.

We're going to go through the four types of *agni* in detail; then we'll talk about ways to support and balance our *agni*.

Balanced Agni

Balanced *agni* is what we are going for! This is one of the goals of an Ayurvedic practice—a strong, balanced, and stable digestive fire.

Signs of balanced *agni* include:

- Hunger at consistent intervals—before breakfast, lunch, and dinner.
- Ability to digest what you are taking in. There is no gas, bloating, discomfort (including cramps), nausea, heaviness, or post-eating fatigue. After eating, you feel light, refuelled, and energized.
- Consistent bowel movements—you are pooping daily without strain, pain, blood, mucous, gas, diarrhea, or constipation. One bowel movement daily is great, one after each meal works too.

---

46   From the *Charaka Samhita, Vimanasthana 6.12.*

Sharp Agni

This is where digestion is intense and creates hyper-metabolism—a lot of hunger but not necessarily a lot of nourishment as the food gets "burned up" in the fire.

Signs of sharp agni include:

- ❑ Desire to frequently eat large amounts of food (hunger is off the charts)
- ❑ Intense craving for sweets
- ❑ Dry throat, lips, and palate (after eating)
- ❑ Heartburn, acid indigestion, hyperacidity, gastritis—various inflammatory conditions can occur
- ❑ Pain in the liver (right side of waist)
- ❑ Hot flashes
- ❑ Hypoglycaemia (a.k.a. low blood sugar)
- ❑ Anger, hate, envy (sharp *agni* is where the term "hangry" comes from)
- ❑ Yellow coating on the tongue
- ❑ A tendency toward diarrhea

What causes sharp *agni*?

- • Sour, salty, oily, or spicy foods
- • Excess exercise
- • Repressed anger
- • An increase in the hot, sharp/penetrating, oily, and spreading qualities

Slow Agni

Also sometimes referred to as dull digestion. This is where digestion is dull or slow and creates hypo-metabolism. This impairment of *agni* makes it hard to get at the nourishment from the food because it takes a long time to break down the food for absorption, if it breaks down the food at all.

Signs of slow *agni* include:

- ❑ Low hunger, low appetite, or loss of appetite
- ❑ Feeling of heaviness in the stomach, nausea, and vomiting
- ❑ Over-salivation, mucous, or edema
- ❑ After eating, a sense of fatigue, lethargy, the desire for sleep (think post-Thanksgiving dinner)
- ❑ Generalized weakness in the body
- ❑ Attachment, greed, and possessiveness
- ❑ Thick white coating on the tongue
- ❑ Slow bowel movements with mucous. Sometimes constipation where it feels like there's too much for it to come out smoothly and easily.

What causes slow *agni*?

- Irregular eating
- Eating often, snacking, or eating before the previous meal is digested
- Cold, heavy foods
- Large quantities of food
- Excessive fasting
- An increase in the heavy, dense, slow, and dull qualities

Variable Agni

This one is where your digestion fluctuates between balanced, sharp, and slow, hence it is referred to as variable. Sometimes people describe it as erratic. Think of it as a fluctuating digestive fire.

Signs of variable *agni* include:

- ❑ Irregular appetite (sometimes you're starving, other times you forget to eat)
- ❑ Gas, bloating, indigestion, abdominal pain, and gurgling in the intestine
- ❑ Dry skin, cracking joints
- ❑ Low back ache
- ❑ Insomnia
- ❑ Anxiety, insecurity, fear
- ❑ Brown/black coating on the tongue
- ❑ A tendency toward constipation or irregular bowel movements (swinging between constipation and diarrhea)

What causes variable *agni*?

- • Emotional stress
- • Irregular eating schedule
- • Eating often, snacking, eating before the previous meal is digested
- • Cold, dry, and raw foods
- • An increase in the cold, mobile, light, dry, and rough qualities

What can I do to support my *agni*?

Now that we know how important *agni* is, here are a few recommendations to help you support, strengthen, and balance your digestive potential:

1. Favour warm cooked foods and avoid ice and cold foods and drinks.

This recommendation has two parts: medicine of addition and medicine of subtraction. *Agni* is fire, and anything cold or icy is going to diminish the fire. For the medicine of addition, add or favour room temperature or warm foods and drinks. This supports and protects the digestive potential, whereas cold (which includes raw) foods make the digestion work harder, which can tire it out.

There is definitely a time and place for some raw food in the diet. That said, if you are noticing that your digestion is variable, sharp, or slow, then subtract cold, raw foods. This is not only a belief held in Ayurveda, it is in other systems as well. My friends who practice Traditional Chinese Medicine notice the same trend. Those with really strong digestive fire are able to maintain a raw food diet for up to five or seven years, and then all of a sudden it becomes really hard to digest without symptoms of gas, bloating, etc.

We want to remember that our *agni* is like a campfire. What would you do to keep your campfire at the perfect size? If you pour ice water on it, what happens to the campfire? It goes out. If you put gasoline on it, what happens? The blaze is huge and out of control, and your eyebrows get singed. We want to be really mindful about what we're putting on our *agni*, which means using discernment before putting anything in our mouths.

So far I've been using food examples, yet it works the same in terms of experiences, emotions, the company we keep ... at every level.

2. Make lunch the largest meal of the day.

A great way to help regulate and strengthen our digestive fire is to make lunchtime the largest meal of the day. Over the lunch hour, our digestion is the strongest. It's also a time of day when we eat before continuing to be mobile and active for the next few hours, which helps our digestion (more on this later). Ideally, we would have lunch anywhere between 11 a.m. and 2 p.m.

Making lunch the largest meal means you're able to digest more foods and you're also able to digest more complicated foods or heavier foods during that time of day with more ease. Whereas, if you try to digest something really heavy in the evening or later at night, your digestive fire isn't as strong, so you might end up with a little bit more indigestion or discomfort than if you were to eat the same thing at lunch.

I recognize that making lunch the biggest meal is more challenging culturally because in the West we tend to make dinnertime the main family meal. This does not mean avoiding a family dinner. Family meals are nourishing for a variety of reasons! The suggestion is to consider the size of the meal at that time of day and maybe make some changes if it would support your digestion and health. The portion size could be a bit bigger at lunch and a bit smaller in the evening. You can still keep other factors the same if you want (like what you are eating, who you are eating with, etc.).

3. Include all SIX tastes[47] in your diet.

Ayurveda has a really brilliant way of working with the taste of food. According to Ayurveda, there are six tastes: sweet, sour, salty, pungent, bitter, and astringent. The different tastes cultivate different qualities, so by eating foods of a certain taste, you are increasing certain qualities. This is one way we can use food to balance our qualities!

1. Sweet

- Associated qualities: cool, heavy, soft, oily, liquid
- Food examples: complex carbs, sweet fruits, grains, root vegetables (potatoes, beets), sugar, honey, dates, milk, cheese, oils, nuts, basil, and meat

2. Sour

- Associated qualities: warm, light, oily, liquid
- Food examples: yogurt, limes, lemons, sour fruits (including tomatoes), alcohol, vinegars, cheese, fermented foods, pickles, garlic, savoury, tamarind

3. Salty

- Associated qualities: warm, wet, heavy, oily
- Food examples: all salts (rock, sea, gypsum, black), celery, tamari, seaweed, soy sauce

---

47   From the *Charaka Samhita, Sutrasthana 1.65.*

4. Pungent

- Associated qualities: warm, dry, light, sharp
- Food examples: jalapeños, chillies, onions, leeks, turnips, kohlrabi, black pepper, cloves, cayenne, ginger, wasabi, radishes, mustard seeds, paprika, hing (asafoetida)

5. Bitter

- Associated qualities: cold, dry, light
- Food examples: green leafy vegetables, eggplant, aloe, goldenseal, fenugreek, myrrh, bitter melon, turmeric, dill, saffron, dandelion, black tea, coffee, sesame seeds, dark chocolate

6. Astringent

- Associated qualities: dry, cold (some sources say light, others say heavy)
- Food examples: raw vegetables, peel of a fruit, unripe bananas, pomegranate peel and seeds, apples, goldenseal, leafy green vegetables, blueberries, cranberries, rye, legumes (especially chickpeas), strong black tea, nutmeg, oregano, fennel, marjoram, rosemary, turmeric, parsley, dill, bay leaf

4. When you eat, focus on your food.

Where we focus our attention is important, as our attention is connected to the fire of the mind. When eating, the best way to digest our food well is to focus on the food. Eat with all your senses by noticing the smells, tastes, colours, and textures. Chew your food thoroughly, until it is liquid. Taste and savour each bite of the food. Remember to breathe while you eat and to pace yourself. I try to take a breath between each fork/spoonful. Have gratitude for your food; we are blessed that we get to nourish ourselves.

When we eat and do something else at the same time, like watch TV, read, or drive our car, we're not actually getting all the nourishment from the food. We lose out on the whole-ness of the experience because we're not being present—not tasting, smelling, seeing—and the distraction of our mind can distract our *agni*.

On a physiological level, when we are engaged in activity, our nervous system shifts out of "rest and digest," which means that the energy is not going toward digestion. Until it does, we don't fully or properly digest our food. If our food isn't well digested, we're not getting all the nourishment we need to maintain our bodies. Focusing on our food as we eat is a really simple way to make a big difference in the quality of our digestion.

5. When hunger arises, EAT.

Hopefully, the urge to eat arises about three to four times per day, at regular intervals. When we have set meal times, this is more likely, and is also what we are trying to culti-vate. When the urge arises, this is a signal that your *agni* has turned on. Hunger is an important sign of *agni* health! When hunger arises, it is important to feed your *agni*. We often sup-press our natural urges, and this is not good for our health. Not responding to this normal healthy signal tells the body we aren't listening to its messages. What happens when we ignore the body? The body stops talking to us.

Of course, sometimes when the urge arises, we cannot respond to it. A great example is getting hungry while you're in a meeting—not much you can do there. However, if it's around a mealtime and the urge to eat arises, it's best to eat.

6. Use ginger to stoke your agni.

The previous recommendation infers that we get hungry; however, sometimes we don't get hungry, which means our *agni* is not ready to receive food. If this happens, or if we are working to train our *agni* for mealtimes, we can use ginger to help enkindle our *agni*. I have three ways I like to do this:

1. Ginger pizzas: These are tasty and effective. Take a piece of ginger root and peel it. Then slice it into thin rounds. Put the thin rounds flat (like they are the pizza crusts) in a glass bowl. Squeeze the juice of a lemon over the ginger slices, then sprinkle sea salt on top. Eat one to two of these *ginger pizzas* about 15 minutes before a meal to turn on the fire in your belly!

2. Ginger tea: This is the simple and portable version. Drink a cup of ginger tea 15 minutes before mealtime. You can use a slice of ginger in hot water, or a ginger tea bag, whichever works for you. I use the tea bags when I'm traveling or if I'm at work.

3. Ginger juice mix: If you have a juicer, this is a very effective option. Juice one ginger root and one turmeric root. Add the juice of half a lemon and a dollop of honey. Mix it together and drink one shot (one ounce) 15 minutes before a meal.

7. Eat until you are no longer hungry.

Somewhere along the way in my life, I picked up the habit of eating until I was full (imagine Thanksgiving dinner). This means that the stomach is so full there might not be enough space in it for the food to mix with the digestive juices to break it down. In Ayurveda school we were invited to "eat until you are no longer hungry." This was a new concept to me. It did two things for me. First, I no longer get "heavy belly after eating." Two, it requires me to pay closer attention while I'm eating. If I'm eating dinner and watching TV, I tend to miss this subtle cue. If I pay attention and stop eating once the hunger subsides, it's the perfect amount that I can digest and still have energy to go for a walk and enjoy my evening.

8. Rest briefly after eating.

Once the meal is complete, take five to ten minutes to rest. If you can, rest while leaning or lying on your left side. This invites the newly ingested food to sit in the part of the stomach that mixes the food with the digestive juices for breakdown. The rest also keeps you in "rest and digest" mode.

9. Make regular exercise and activity a priority.

Being active is important. The more sedentary we are the weaker our digestive fire becomes. When we are active and keep the body moving and circulating, it really helps to stoke the fire.

Another interesting aspect of this one is that many people find they do a lot of mental-emotional processing when they move their bodies, which tells me that movement is not only good for biological digestion but also mental-emotional digestion. Movement helps us clear our channels!

I see this in my yoga classes all the time. A lot of people come to practice, and this gives them an opportunity to digest the events of the day. If they skip their practice for a while, then their body and mind get boggy; they can feel that things aren't clear and flowing. We'll talk more about what that bogginess is in the next section.

Years ago I read Swami Rama's autobiography. In it, he talks about the importance of taking 100 steps after eating. It is something that has stuck in our household, especially since we got a dog. After dinner we go for 100 steps, and it's a wonderful way to get the food digesting and the nutrition flowing. It also helps gravity move things in the right direction.

10. Maintain a daily routine.

One of the best ways to keep *agni* strong is to have a basic daily routine. This does not mean that every moment of your day is pre-planned (unless you want that), it means having a basic structure that lets your digestion know when to turn on and when to turn off. When things are irregular, the *agni* doesn't know when to be ready and when to rest. This affects our hunger, our energy, and our stability.

Start with making the following five things consistent:

1. Wake time: get up around the same time every day. Ideally, before the sun rises—we'll talk more about this later in the book.

2. Breakfast: have breakfast between 7 a.m. and 9 a.m.

3. Lunch: eat lunch as your biggest meal between 11 a.m. and 2 p.m.

4. Dinner: have dinner between 5:30 p.m. and 7 p.m.

5. Bedtime: go to bed around the same time each day.

In between these parts of your routine, work, play, have fun, and live your life. Eating at around the same time each day is a huge support to your digestion. Your body thrives on this type of routine, and your *agni* knows when to fire up and when to rest.

When there's no routine at all, the digestion is one of the first things to become impaired. Think about when you travel: your routine is different, and most people get hungry at weird times. You crave a lot of sugar and refined junk foods, and then arrive at your destination tired and constipated, which makes you anxious and cranky.

11. Stay hydrated.

It is important that you drink enough clean water over the course of the day for your system to maintain balance. When the body gets dehydrated, the digestive system gets nervous about turning the fire on. After all, if you put a fire in a cardboard box, what happens? The fire will consume the box. The stomach requires enough fluid to secrete mucous to protect the stomach, as well as the liquid medium to dissolve the food in (which helps to break down food). If you're dehydrated, you might have fire, but your body won't use it.

Dry skin and mouth and tongue, dizziness, headaches, constipation, or scanty (or missing) menstruation and urination are all signs of dehydration. The guideline for drinking water is eight 250mL glasses per day. That said, in Ayurveda we know that some folks need more, and others need less. If you need help with this, find an Ayurvedic Counsellor to guide you.

There's another aspect to this recommendation, which is making sure the water you drink is actually being absorbed into your tissues. Ever drink a lot of water and still feel thirsty? It's like you pee all the fluid out and none of it soaks in? If this happens to you, it might be helpful to use **boiled water** instead of regular water, or to add one serving of **homemade healthy hydration drink** (see recipes below) to your fluid intake.

Boiled Water

Each morning I fill a large pot with water. Then I put it on the stove top and turn the burner on high to bring the water to a boil. Boil the water until ¼ (25%) of the water is evaporated, then turn off the burner. Boiling the water changes its qualities—it adds more warmth and lightness to it, making the water easier for your body to absorb. Then once it cools down a little, this is the water I drink for the day. I'll even use boiled water in the kettle and warm it back up.

Homemade Healthy Hydration Drink

This hydration drink helps your body absorb the water you drink. I use it in the summertime when I'm dehydrated, or when I'm very active like at the gym. My friend Staraya McKinstry-Robinson (a wonderful Ayurvedic Practitioner in the US) shared this recipe with our class, and I have passed it forward ever since.

1. Take 3 cups of water (that's three of the eight you need daily ☺).

2. Add the juice of a lime or lemon (use lime if you run hot, use lemon if you run cold).

3. Add sea/rock salt (I do three grinds from my grinder).

4. Add 1 tablespoon of maple syrup.

5. Stir and drink.

The salt increases water absorption into the cells. The maple syrup adds nutrition to the plasma (the plasma is our sap, and maple syrup is the sap of a tree—like increases like). The citrus boosts the *agni* so it gets well digested. I take this and split the 3 cups into two water bottles—one for the morning, and one for the afternoon.

12. Choose a supportive eating environment.

Ayurveda not only believes that what you eat is important, it also emphasizes that HOW and WHERE you eat are important because what you do and where you are affects your nervous system (remember "active fight or flight" and "rest and digest"?). Here are some considerations. Even if you can't do them all, see which ones you can do and start there. Remember that every step you take in the direction of your health is a step in the direction of your health!

- Eat in a calm and peaceful environment: think "romantic meal" even if you are the only one eating.

- Sit to eat: standing shifts the gears of your nervous system out of "rest and digest."

- Eat in a clean space: clear the table of all non-essentials before sitting to eat; this calms the nerves.

- Have something nice to look at: perhaps a plant, some flowers, art that appeals to you, or a window where you can look outside. Our dining room table looks outside and has our aerogarden on it. I love to look outside and check on my herbs while I eat. It relaxes me.

- Be present and mindful: notice where you are, who you are with, and what you are doing. Being present while eating allows you to enjoy your food more (and the company or scenery) and digest it better.

- Take a break: step away from working, texting, checking emails, etc. to eat. It's amazing how quickly any of these things can shift our gears into the stress response.

13. Have an herbal tea after eating.

Herbal teas are wonderful digestive aids. If you tend to get gassy, bloated, or feel heavy in the tummy after eating, try ginger or turmeric tea. If you tend to get acidic (like acid reflux or burning sensations) after eating, try mint or fennel tea.

What Happens If My *Agni* Is Impaired (Variable, Sharp, Slow)?

When the digestive fire is impaired, not only are we unable to get nourishment from our food, but also the part that we don't fully digest becomes a problem.

Ama—*metabolic waste*

In Sanskrit we call this undigested material *ama*, which translates to "metabolic waste products." *Ama* is thick, sticky, and heavy. It does not move through our system well; instead, it causes clogs in our channels and tissues.

One view of the human body is as a series of channels. We have channels, or pipes, for all sorts of things. A few examples include:

- arteries and veins to circulate the blood and plasma
- lymphatic channels to circulate the lymph and immune cells
- gastrointestinal tract allows for the intake of food and the elimination of wastes from the bowels
- channels for muscle, bone, breath, emotions, and even thoughts

Our entire body-mind is a series of channels that allows all sorts of stuff to flow through unless they are clogged by *ama*.

When we are unable to digest our food, emotions, thoughts, and experiences, a thick sticky residue begins to build up in our system. This affects our body's ability to circulate nourishment, to build healthy tissues, and to easily eliminate wastes. It also depletes the body-mind of its vital energy, of its *prana*. All of a sudden, more resources need to be allocated to cleansing, clearing, and managing this *ama*. The more *ama* that builds up, the less energetic, vibrant, and healthy we feel. If there's enough *ama* in our system, we experience pain or fatigue.

> *Ama* is the root of disease. In Ayurveda, we prevent disease by strengthening *agni*, so there is no *ama* to cause disease.

Vagbhata describes *ama* in the following ways:

> Those persons who indulge in incompatible/unhealthy foods and overeating will become victims of *ama*, which produces symptoms similar to those of poison.

> Foods which are hard to digest, dry, cold, disliked; those which cause constipation or burning sensation, which are dirty (rotten, polluted); drinking large amounts of water; foods which are mainly liquid, these taken at improper time; foods and drinks taken by a person who is afflicted with lust, anger, greed, jealousy, shyness, grief, fear, and hunger, are also going to produce *ama* in the body.[48]

Most people have a little bit of *ama*, as there's always something somewhere that wasn't digested 100% perfectly. But when the digestive fire remains strong over time, it is able to digest or break down any *ama* that has accumulated in the system. The more *ama* in the system, the harder the *agni* has

---

48   From the *Ashtanga Samgraha, Sutrasthana 11.7–8.*

to work to digest what we ingest, as well as the *ama*. That's a heavy load.

How do I know if I have ama?

We know that *ama* builds when we are unable to digest whatever it is that we take into the body-mind. Again, everyone has some *ama*, and your body is designed to get rid of a certain amount of it. It's when we end up with an accumulation that it begins to cause problems in the systems of the body.

Signs of *ama* in the body:

- ❑ White coated tongue, especially in the morning
- ❑ Foul smell—breath, body, and bowel movements (one or all of these)
- ❑ Sticky stool—it stains the toilet bowl when you flush
- ❑ Constipation
- ❑ Poor appetite
- ❑ Congestion and heaviness
- ❑ Fatigue and achy body
- ❑ Feel tired and lethargic during the day—especially late afternoon, even though you're getting enough sleep
- ❑ Vague aches and pains or a general lack of well-being
- ❑ Low vitality, a lack of motivation, no "zest for life"
- ❑ Mind feels cloudy, unclear, "spaced out," or foggy

Again, we all have some *ama*, and our body is able to take care of that. With a little bit, we would only show mild signs. We want to watch for an accumulation of *ama*, the amount that our body can't take care of naturally, because that leads to getting sick. As the signs show more, or build up, then we need to focus on building our *agni* in order to digest the *ama* that is in our system and reduce the production of more *ama*. Our body is always giving us information, and Ayurveda wants to help us understand its language so we know what it's trying to tell us.

How can I prevent *ama*?

Now that we know what *ama* is and does, here are some recommendations to help you prevent *ama* from forming in your system:

1. Strengthen and support your agni.

When *agni* is strong and stable, we don't produce *ama*. And when it's strong enough, it can digest the *ama*. A strong digestive fire is key to getting rid of *ama*.

2. Reduce anything "undigestible."

If you know you don't digest something well or at all (think sensitivities and allergies), stop consuming it. As soon as you eat it, *ama* is happening.

3. Avoid overconsumption.

This goes along with supporting your *agni*; however, when you notice that you have *ama*, it's time to lighten the load on the digestion. Eat smaller portions and let go of snacks. Create space for digestion to take place. Allow enough room in your stomach in order for the hydrochloric acid to mix in with the food particles in the water medium. Then you need room in order for the churning to happen and for the breakdown of that food to take place. In your life there needs to be room between things happening for you to process what's going on, for you to integrate, and for you to fully digest and assimilate what's happening to you.

4. Choose simple, light, and easy-to-digest foods.

Anything that's heavy (foods, experiences, emotions) and in large quantities (another form of heavy) is going to be hard to digest and results in an accumulation of *ama*. When you feel heavy, or heavy is happening in your life, then it's time to eat light foods. Some examples are: chicken or fish instead of steak; soup instead of pizza; or steamed veggies instead of veggies sautéed in oil. A few ways that I simplify are making three dishes instead of five for dinner, skipping sauces or dressings (they often have many ingredients), or letting go of heavy foods like wheat and dairy until my digestion is back on track.

5. Reduce fast food, processed food, foods with additives (if you can't pronounce it, don't eat it) leftovers, and canned and frozen foods.

The additional processing and preservation can alter the food, making it harder to digest, and from hard-to-digest we get *ama*. As much as possible, we are invited to eat fresh local foods, simply prepared. It's not always possible—trust me, I get it. However, when *ama* is building up in our system, we need to put some extra effort into our food choices—it really does matter and make a difference. Pull out your slow cooker or electric pressure cooker or go to the simple and easy recipes you have on hand.

6. Use basic food combining.

Mixing different foods together is a science, not only for the taste combinations, but for the effects on our digestion. When our digestion is strong, our *agni* can figure out how to digest pretty much anything. When it isn't, food combining becomes an important part of resetting and strengthening the digestive fire. I was introduced to this concept during a time when my digestion was very poor, so this was a powerful and useful tool for me. I still use the basic principles in my day-to-day cooking.

Here are food combinations to AVOID, as they are *ama* producing:

- Milk and fish

- Eggs and dairy (for my frittata I use almond milk instead)

- Nuts with vegetables or beans

- Sour fruits (lemon, lime, orange) with dairy (if it curdles outside your body, it also curdles inside your stomach)

- More than two grains together (watch out for complicated gluten-free flour blends that have many grains mixed together)

There are many other food combining guidelines in Ayurveda, and I know that there are other approaches to food combining separate from Ayurveda. These five will get you started.

Along with the above recommendations, there are a few things we can do to get rid of the daily accumulation of *ama* in our system, which brings more stability to our sense organs and balance in our qualities.

1. Scrape your tongue first thing in the morning.

As you sleep, your body works to clean and detoxify your system. Any *ama* it finds is moved to the gastrointestinal tract, from the tongue all the way down to the rectum, for elimination. Isn't it awesome how your body knows what it's doing? Knowing this, it is a good idea to scrape your tongue in the morning when you wake up. Make sure you look at what comes off—your body is trying to communicate with you! The colour, thickness, and amount are all signs of how your digestion is.

2. Drink a cup of warm (or room temperature) water.

After you scrape your tongue and brush your teeth, drink a cup of warm (or room temperature) water to hydrate the body and help flush the *ama* from your throat down and out through the rectum, which is the natural channel of elimination for the gastrointestinal tract.

3. Practice nasal rinsing using a neti pot and salt water.

This technique is known as *jala neti*, in Sanskrit. *Neti* is a wonderful technique to rinse the nasal passages, clearing them in order to facilitate nasal breathing.

I remember the first time I tried this—it freaked me right out. It actually freaked me out enough to want to quit my 200-hour yoga teacher training ... until I did it and I breathed so deep and clear that I've done it every day since, and that was in 2004.

Neti is not recommended if you have a nosebleed, or too

much of the cold, heavy, thick, slimy/sticky, or liquid qualities already present in your head. I tend to be dry, so *neti* works really well for me daily. However, those who tend to be more cold, heavy, thick, slimy, and sticky might find that *neti* clears their nose for a bit, then the feeling of heavy, thick, slimy, and sticky comes back even more—remember, like increases like. No technique works for everyone all of the time. If you have too much of the cold, heavy, thick, slimy, and sticky qualities, consider a dry sauna instead of a nasal rinse.

Fill your *neti* pot with clean warm water and sea salt. The sea salt measurement is about ½–1 teaspoon sea salt for each cup of water. The idea is to adjust the water to the salinity (or saltiness) of your own tears. If you ever try it without salt, it will create a burning sensation in your nose. Ironically, the same thing will happen if there's too much salt. Like Goldilocks, we're looking for a balanced place of "just right."

Once the pot and salt water are set up, allow the water to flow through the nasal passages with gravity. It is not recommended to sniff the water up into the nose or to use any forceful means that can damage sensitive nasal tissues. You can add a bit of baking soda (half the amount of the salt) to the mix if your nasal tissues are very dry or sensitive.

For this one, **I strongly recommend getting instruction from someone with experience using a *neti* pot.** The way you position your head and body makes a difference in terms of getting the water to flow through the proper channels in your head—in one nostril and out the other, instead of in one nostril and down the throat.

4. Drink CCF tea.

CCF tea stands for cumin, coriander, and fennel tea. Cumin, coriander, and fennel are three herbs that boost the *agni* and, at the same time, eat up *ama*.

To make this tea, mix equal portions of cumin seeds, coriander seeds, and fennel seeds in a clean glass jar with a lid. When you are ready to make the tea itself, use 1 teaspoon of the seed mixture in 1–2 cups of hot water. You can strain it, then drink it, and you can even eat the seeds (they are food).

Note: This recommendation does not make sense for anyone with an allergy or sensitivity to cumin, coriander, or fennel. In that case, feel free to omit the seed(s) you are allergic to and make your tea with the ones that are safe for you to consume.

5. Meditate daily.

Ama not only builds up in the channels of the body, it builds up in the mental-emotional channels too. Meditation is a tool to digest what is in the mental-emotional channels, from experiences to *ama*, and to get that channel flowing freely again. There are many approaches to meditation, all of them beneficial for clearing the channels of the heart-mind.

One of the simplest meditation techniques is breath awareness meditation. Find a comfortable seat (if you aren't comfortable, you'll be constantly distracted by the discomfort) and settle in. Soften your gaze. If it feels safe, close your eyes. Let your body relax and focus on the natural flow of your breath. Natural breath means that you watch your breath as it is; no need to change it by making it longer or slowing it down, simply notice your breath. Then pay attention, as full of attention as you can, to your breathing. Notice the in-breaths (known as inhalations) and the out-breaths (known as exhalations). Notice if your breath makes sound or is quiet—listen to your breath. Notice where in your body the breath creates movement—feel your breath.

Learn from a teacher if you can—it is more valuable than you can imagine. I tried meditating on my own for the first five years. Then I stumbled upon a teacher and made more progress in one year with him than I had in the previous five years on my own. What I learned from my teacher was that meditation wasn't what I thought it was. I wasn't making progress because I was confused about what the practice was. It's a practice of focus, presence, patience, and compassion. Having a guide to help you through the vast terrain of the mind is immensely valuable—especially if you have mental *ama* to digest. Find a teacher and begin getting the clogs out of your mental pipes.

6. Alternate nostril breathing.

This is a yoga technique that helps get *ama* out of the channels of the breath and mind. It also engages and harmonizes both hemispheres of the brain, bringing the whole nervous system back into balance. This is another technique that I recommend you learn from an experienced yoga teacher or Ayurvedic practitioner.

Find a comfortable seated position. Remember that sitting in a chair is completely legal—especially if it makes you more comfortable. Take a few moments to become aware of your body, breath, emotions, mind, and heart. Focus on your breath and allow the breath to flow naturally.

Using the right hand, bring the index and middle fingers of the right hand to the base of the thumb. Extend the R thumb and R ring and pinky fingers. This position is known as *Vishnu mudra*. Bring your R hand to your face. The R thumb will gently close the R nostril, and the R ring and pinky fingers will gently close the L nostril.

Now for the technique itself. These instructions describe one round:

- Use the R thumb to gently close the R nostril, and inhale through the L nostril.
- Switch the fingers after the inhalation so the R ring and pinky gently close the L nostril, and exhale through the R nostril.
- Inhale in the R nostril.
- Switch the fingers and exhale through the L nostril.

As you practice, keep the breath gentle, easy, and smooth. Remember not to hold or force the breath. Be gentle and kind to yourself as you practice.

Begin by trying five rounds, then go back to natural breathing. Over time, work your way up to 15 minutes daily. I set a timer so I don't have to watch the clock, and I find that works really well for me.

Agni and *Ama* Conclusion

Our digestive fire (*agni*) is important because without it we don't benefit from the nourishment we take in. Not only do we lose nourishment if our digestion is impaired, we have a buildup of *ama* in our channels that can clog our pipes.

In the next section we're going to talk more about how the nourishment becomes our tissues. We'll get to the BIG WHY of nourishment as a pillar of health.

CHAPTER 6

BUILDING HEALTHY TISSUES

The nourishment we ingest, digest, and absorb becomes our tissues, known as *dhatu* in Sanskrit. The goal is to have proper tissue formation, in the proper amount, in the appropriate places. When this doesn't happen, a wide variety of diseases can occur, such as lipoma, fibroid, blood clot, endometriosis, or cancer. All of these are examples of tissue imbalance where the tissues are not forming properly, so we end up with an improper amount of tissue or tissue in the wrong places.

Consider a uterine fibroid as an example. The uterus is meant to be a hollow organ, and yet the fibroid grows and fills that space. It is not proper tissue formation; there's too much tissue, and it's not in the right place.

From the Ayurvedic view, we need to find balance in order to optimize our health. Balanced tissues are very important for the maintenance of the physical body. It is also important for the mind, because the body is the container for the mind. I talked earlier about how the body-mind is a system of channels. These tissues are those very channels! If we want good flow through the channels, through our pipes, then we need good tissues (strong pipes).

The quantity and quality of our tissues is affected by the quality of our digestion, as well as the quality and quantity of the food we eat. There are a few different things that can happen.

The *quality of the food* determines the quality of the tissues. Good-quality food that you can digest produces healthy and strong tissues. Poor-quality food produces poor-quality tissues. This is where "you are what you eat" comes from … although in Ayurveda we say "you are what you digest" because we are obsessed with *agni*.

The *quantity of the food* determines the quantity of the tissues. If you eat a high quantity (a lot of food), you are able to build more tissues. If you do not eat enough for your metabolism, then you will not build enough tissues. We see both of these in our modern-day context actually: folks who are overweight (too much tissue) and folks who are underweight (not enough tissue). Neither is healthy.

Regardless of the quality and quantity of food, if our *digestion* is impaired, we produce a higher quantity of *ama* (more clogs in the pipes) and a lower quantity and quality of body tissue (weak pipes). The ideal situation is strong and balanced digestion, which leads to minimal *ama* and the proper amount of tissues (good quantity) that are strong and resilient (good quality).

According to Ayurveda, there are seven main tissue types that develop from the nourishment we consume and digest. They are "all pervading," which means they are everywhere in your body. This makes these particular tissues fundamentally important because they are everywhere in your system! Although tissue production is an ongoing process for the biology, the way Ayurveda describes tissue production is that the tissues get built in order, each tissue taking five days to build: plasma and lymph, blood, muscle, adipose, bone, marrow, and reproductive.

Tissue Production – Ayurvedic View

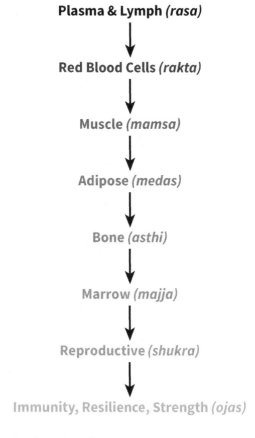

Plasma & Lymph *(rasa)*

Red Blood Cells *(rakta)*

Muscle *(mamsa)*

Adipose *(medas)*

Bone *(asthi)*

Marrow *(majja)*

Reproductive *(shukra)*

Immunity, Resilience, Strength *(ojas)*

The catch, then, is that the latter tissues get built only if there is enough nourishment left that far along in the process. Each tissue takes five days to build, so to rebuild all seven levels of tissues takes 40 days (which is six weeks).

Let's look more closely at these seven critical tissues.

First Tissue—Plasma and Lymph (*Rasa*)

The plasma is the nourishing fluid of the body and the main component of the blood (forming about 55%). It transports nutrients to every cell through the cardiovascular system. The cardiovascular system consists of the heart (the pump), arteries (channels that move blood from the heart to the cells and tissues), capillaries (channels where nutrients go into cells from the blood and wastes move out of cells into the blood), veins (channels that return the blood back to the heart), and blood that circulates through these channels. Without good-quality plasma (the right thickness and amount) and good circulation of the plasma, the body lacks nourishment.

The lymph is the immune fluid of the body, and it drains the waste products and unwanted materials out of the body. Some of the plasma from the blood drains into lymphatic capillaries and becomes "lymph." Lymph is what we call the fluid that moves through the lymphatic vessels to lymph nodes where this fluid gets cleansed of waste materials. The waste materials are moved out of the body via the regular waste elimination channels, which are discussed in the next chapter. Once the fluid is cleaned, the clean lymph goes back into cardiovascular circulation at the heart, where it becomes plasma again. The white blood cells found in the blood are also part of the lymphatic system, as they are fighting and removing infectious agents that have entered into the body.

Together, the plasma and lymph create an interconnected systemic circulation that nourishes every cell and removes waste from every cell of your body. In Sanskrit, they are called *rasa*, which means "essence," "sap," and "nutritive fluid."

The villain of Plasma and Lymph Land is stagnation, a lack of flow or circulation. My teacher Dr. Claudia says that when there is stagnation, 100% of the time there is pain in that area. So if you have pain somewhere, you have stagnation, which means a flow issue through those pipes. Where there is stagnation, the nourishment is reduced, and the waste elimination too. This means that *ama* builds up and the discomfort/pain increases.

Recommendations for Plasma and Lymph

1. Drink enough water.

Our plasma and lymph are fluids and are affected by the amount of water we consume. We need to drink enough water to keep our plasma and lymph full and fluid. Drinking soda, coffee, tea, juice, and other beverages doesn't count as drinking water. Drinking pure clean water is really important for health because it forms the basis of this nourishing tissue— the tissue that nourishes all the other tissues! If you have dry skin and mouth and tongue, dizziness, headaches, constipation, or scanty menstruation and urination (or it's missing), these are signs of dehydration, and you may need to drink more water. The guideline for drinking water is eight 250mL glasses per day. That said, in Ayurveda we know that some folks need more, and others need less. If you need help with this, find an Ayurvedic Counsellor to guide you.

There's another aspect to this recommendation, which is making sure the water you drink is actually being absorbed into your tissues. Ever drink a lot of water and you're still thirsty? It's like you pee all the fluid out and none of it soaks in? If this happens to you, it might be helpful to use **boiled water** instead of regular water, or to add one serving of **homemade healthy hydration drink** (recipes below) to your fluid intake.

Boiled Water

Each morning I fill a large pot with water. Then I put it on the stove top and turn the burner on high to bring the water to a boil. Boil the water until ¼ (25%) of the water is evaporated, then turn off the burner. Boiling the water changes its qualities—it adds more warmth and lightness to it, making the water easier for your body to absorb. Then once it cools down a little, this is the water I drink for the day. I'll even use boiled water in the kettle and warm it back up.

Homemade Healthy Hydration Drink

This hydration drink helps your body absorb the water you drink. I use it in the summertime when I'm dehydrated, or when I'm very active like at the gym. My friend Staraya McKinstry-Robinson (a wonderful Ayurvedic Practitioner in the US) shared this recipe with our class, and I have passed it forward ever since.

1. Take 3 cups of water (that's three of the eight you need daily ☺).

2. Add the juice of a lime or lemon (use lime if you run hot, use lemon if you run cold).

3. Add sea/rock salt (I do three grinds from my grinder).

4. Add 1 tablespoon of maple syrup.

5. Stir and drink.

The salt increases water absorption into the cells. The maple syrup adds nutrition to the plasma (the plasma is our sap, and maple syrup is the sap of a tree—like increases like). The citrus boosts the *agni* so it gets well digested. I take this and split the 3 cups into two water bottles—one for the morning, and one for the afternoon.

2. Move your body daily to prevent stagnation.

This might mean taking a 20-minute walk, a bike ride, or a yoga class. The human body is designed to move, and it needs to move daily for a minimum of 20 minutes. Unlike the cardio-vascular system (heart, arteries, and veins), which circulates the plasma using the heart as its pump, the lymphatic system (lymph vessels, nodes, and ducts) has no pump and requires movement for circulation. So where we don't move regularly, our lymph does not circulate, and it stagnates. And as mentioned earlier, 100% of the time where there is stagnation, there is pain. The expression is "move it or lose it," and it is true on so many levels! It is really important to move your body every day. And the cardiovascular system also benefits greatly from daily movement—just sayin'!

3. Practice dry brushing.

This is done with a raw silk glove before taking a shower or bath. The entire body benefits from this technique. Some sources recommend daily, others weekly, and others seasonally (this is a great practice for the spring season). This is a helpful practice if your lymphatic and circulatory systems tend to be sluggish (if you have stagnation), or if your skin gets itchy. Be careful with dry or aging skin, as well as with the face and genital regions. If you have super dry skin, it's best to skip this.

For dry brushing, begin at your feet and work your way up the body. Use long strokes (back and forth) across the long bones, and circular motions (round and round) at the joints, abdomen, low back, and breasts.

Note: Remember to wash your raw silk gloves regularly and hang them dry.

4. Eat white foods.

Think potatoes, cauliflower, zucchini, onions, garlic, bananas, and dairy. These are dense and nutritious foods, which nourish the plasma. Remember, in order for the food to be nourishing, your *agni* has to be able to digest it!

Second Tissue—Blood (*Rakta*)

Red blood cells are the second tissue developed from the nourishment you consume. The red blood cells have the function of "life giving," which makes sense given that they carry oxygen to provide energy to every single one of your cells. The red blood cells are mixed with your plasma and are circulated through the cardiovascular system.

The cardiovascular system integrates not only with the lymphatic system (as described above), but also with the respiratory system. Your respiratory system includes your breathing channels—your nose, bronchus (windpipe), and lungs. The lungs take in air, which includes oxygen. The blood moves from the heart to the lungs, where through pulmonary capillaries, the oxygen from the air attaches to the red blood cells in the blood, and any gas wastes move from the blood into the air. This oxygenated blood returns to the heart to be circulated systemically through the cardiovascular system.

In the Ayurvedic teachings, the cardiovascular and pulmonary systems are viewed as one functional unit. Without oxygenating the blood (which happens in the lungs), there's no point in circulating the blood. Likewise, without having a way to circulate the oxygenated blood to all the cells, there isn't much point in breathing.

Without the plasma as a nutrient-delivery system, there would be no way to deliver the oxygen to the cells in the rest of your body. I appreciate the brilliance of the order of the tissue development.

Some of the more common challenges in the blood tissue are circulation issues, excess clotting, or anemia (lack of red blood cells). All of these affect the blood's ability to deliver oxygen to the cells, which hinders their function.

Recommendations for Blood

1. Eat green and red foods.

Green leafy vegetables like kale, chard, broccoli, spinach, and asparagus are high in iron and minerals. This strengthens the blood. These veggies also support liver function, and since the liver cleanses the blood, this supports both. Red foods like beets, pomegranate, and berries (cherries, cranberries, raspberries, blackberries, blueberries, strawberries) are great to support cardiovascular and lymphatic circulation. Try to eat green and red foods daily.

2. Drink nettle tea.

Stinging nettle is a North American plant that is very high in minerals, especially iron. A cup of nettle tea a day has helped many of my iron-deficient clients raise their iron count, which means they also raise their energy levels. This is a particularly great tea in the summertime when the nettle plant grows in abundance.

There are other mineral-dense rich foods as well that support the blood tissue, like liver, meat, fish, tofu, eggs, pulses, beans, nuts, seeds, apricots, prunes, raisins, molasses, whole grains (like rice), and dark leafy veggies (which we already talked about).

Note: This is an area where I believe working with a live practitioner is most helpful. If you are noticing signs and symptoms of low energy that might be iron deficiency, it's important to get the proper testing done to make sure you actually know what's happening so you can address the root issue.

3. Practice mindful three-part breathing.

The above recommendations encourage strong blood tissue, this one is about making sure you have enough oxygen coming into the body for the red blood cells to deliver to all your cells.

A great technique for oxygenation is the "three-part breath." It's diaphragmatic, thoracic, and clavicular (collarbone) breathing, which means it uses the whole lung for breathing (lower, middle, and upper lobes of the lungs). Many folks are shallow breathers, which is connected to our "fight or flight" stress response, and only use a small portion of the lungs, which means they are not getting as much oxygen as they could be. When this happens we end up feeling tired and lethargic. The three-part breath was designed to use as much of your lungs for breath as you can, to bring in as much oxygen as you can.

Breathing is best learned from a qualified yoga teacher or breath expert. The basic technique of three-part breathing begins with finding a comfortable position; most people prefer seated or reclined. Bring one hand to your low belly, below your navel, and the other hand to your low ribs. As you begin the inhalation (breathing in), draw the breath deep into the lower lungs (diaphragmatic). When the breath moves into the lower lungs, toward the belly, you might feel your belly move toward the hand that is on the belly. After practicing this a few times, on the in-breath fill the belly, then allow the ribs to expand outward to fill the middle lungs (thoracic). As the breath moves into the lungs, you'll feel the ribs move into the hand that is positioned on the ribs. Finally, breathe into the belly and ribs, and all the way up into the collarbones (clavicles) to fill the upper lungs (clavicular). This uses the full lung and rib cage for breathing, and this type of breathing supports oxygenation and circulation. The exhalation (breathing out) might be from the top down or bottom up, depending on which feels better to you.

Third Tissue—Muscle (*Mamsa*)

The third tissue to be built is muscle. Muscle tissue is our "meat," and it provides us with connection, strength, and movement. Its function is to cover the body and provide a layer of protection. There are three types of muscle found in the body.

The first is cardiac muscle. It's the type of muscle that makes up your heart and is part of your cardiovascular system. What makes this muscle unique is that it self-regulates—it contracts and releases on its own, no matter what. And really, thank goodness for that! Could you imagine staying up at night to make sure your heart kept beating?

The second is known as smooth muscle. This type of muscle lines the organs of the gastrointestinal tract. It creates a wave-like movement known as "peristalsis," which moves the food down the esophagus (which is the channel from your throat to your stomach), and through the small and large intestines. It also creates the churning movement in the stomach that mixes the food with the stomach juices (go *agni*!). Smooth muscle also lines the urinary bladder and uterus so they can stretch when needed. Think of how the body allows you to hold urine or support a baby, contracting when it's time to release. Most of this type of muscular work is governed by the nervous system and happens automatically. I call it "auto-magic" because if every time I swallowed my food I had to focus on contracting all the muscles it takes to get my food digested and eliminated, I'm not sure I'd make it!

The third type of muscle is called skeletal. These connect the bones to each other and, in working with the bones (which act as levers), help us to move our limbs and various body parts. This type of muscle is what is called voluntary, which means it is under conscious control. We choose to walk, run, lift weights, or do yoga.

Ayurveda describes the muscle as connected to the skin, which is our main protective barrier against pathogens (diseases) in the outside world. And like the other tissues, muscle permeates our entire system; we have muscles everywhere. Our muscle tissue is fed by our blood and plasma.

Recommendations for Muscle

1. Eat grains, nuts, meats, and legumes.

These are the foods that are most nourishing and building for the muscle tissue. Making sure you have the right amount of these protein-rich foods allows your body to build strong muscles.

2. Exercise your muscles.

Lifting weights and prioritizing movement-based activities that engage the muscle tissue keeps the muscles healthy and strong, and nutrients (food) and energy (oxygen) flowing through these channels.

3. Relax your muscles.

We want to work the muscles, and we also need them to know how to relax. A lot of us get tight muscles, and if they can't relax (untighten), it causes pain and discomfort. Tight muscles are often connected to our "active fight or flight" stress response. Remember that pain is a sign of stagnation, which means that something is blocking the flow through this channel. This can be constriction (like a tight muscle) or inflammation (think "itis"—bursitis, tendonitis, etc.). Either way, it involves pain, and that's how your body tells you that something isn't flowing well.

Learning to relax the muscles reduces constriction and inflammation, which reduces pain. You can learn to relax using breathing, stretching, meditation (all of these are part of yoga), mindfulness, listening to relaxing music, being in nature, or watching a funny movie. Think about what relaxes you, and make sure you take the time to do this for yourself on a regular basis.

Fourth Tissue—Adipose (*Meda*)

The fourth tissue that gets built is adipose, or fat. In the West, there is a tendency toward "fat phobia." We don't realize that there is great benefit to having the proper amount of healthy adipose tissue. Healthy adipose has many functions. It provides lubrication (so things run smoothly—think of smooth flow through the pipes), insulation (so we don't freeze and get sick, no one wants frozen pipes!), and energy reserves. The key is *healthy* adipose, which means eating healthy fats. In the West, we have access to an abundance of unhealthy fats, which are inexpensive and easy to find. This is why we have many obesity-based diseases, caused by boggy and sluggish flow through the channels.

Recommendations for Adipose

1. Eat healthy fats.

Healthy fats come from nuts, seeds, avocados, fatty fish (like salmon, tuna, mackerel, sardines), vegetable oils (olive, sunflower, peanut, sesame, coconut, etc.), and *ghee* (clarified butter). Avoid foods with trans fats; these are the harmful fats that create poor quality and excess quantity of adipose.

2. Keep your agni strong.

One of the main reasons we end up with excess adipose tissue is because our *agni* (digestive potential) is impaired. When our body produces *ama* (clogs), one of the places our body stores these toxins is in the adipose tissue to "insulate" it from damaging the rest of the body. Keep your *agni* strong by eating at regular mealtimes, eating good-quality nourishing foods, and letting go of snacking.

Fifth Tissue—Bone (*Asthi*)

The fifth tissue is bone. Our skeleton serves multiple functions: it provides structure to the body, protection to vital organs, sturdy attachment points for the muscles (without this, no matter how strong your muscles are, there would be no movement), and storage for minerals. Our bones provide us with a sense of stability in our being. The skeleton is at the essence of standing tall and moving forward.

Some of the challenges we see with the bone tissue is weakness, deformity, and degeneration.

Recommendations for Bone

1. Consume bone broth.

We learned earlier that like increases like, so if we want to build bone tissue, then we benefit from consuming bone tissue. One of the most accessible forms is bone broth. When I have time, I make my own (I use the slow cooker function of my Instant Pot to cook it overnight), which is the ideal. However, when I don't have time to make my own, I buy organic chicken broth that doesn't have a bunch of extra additives that I can't pronounce. I have a rule that if I can't pronounce the word, I don't put it in my body—and I practice the Sanskrit language, so that says something.

2. Include weight-bearing exercise in your routine.

These are exercises that encourage your bones to strengthen against the pull of gravity. It includes things like weight lifting, walking, hiking, jogging, stair climbing, dancing, and aerobics. Activities that are not as weight-bearing include swimming and bicycling.

3. Reduce your consumption of refined white sugar.

Refined white sugar has no vitamins and minerals, which means it contains no nutritional value. Sugar absorbs quickly into the bloodstream and alters the pH of the body, making it more acidic. To buffer against this internal acidity, the body uses calcium, which it takes from the bones. Sugar also reduces our phosphorus, vitamin D, zinc, and magnesium—not just our calcium. Where we can reduce sugar, our body is stronger and healthier, right down to the bones!

If you do need some sweetener in your life, consider honey, maple syrup, jaggery (raw cane sugar), or stevia.

Sixth Tissue—Marrow (*Majja*)

The sixth tissue that gets built is marrow, deep in the bones. The health of this tissue is strongly associated with nervous function, in particular the myelin sheath. In Ayurveda, both of these tissues perform the function of filling the hollow spaces. The marrow refers to bone marrow, which fills the hollow cavities of our long bones and produces blood cells (both red and white). Nerve cells make up our nervous system, which includes our brain, spinal cord, and all the nerve fibres that connect the spinal cord to all the organs, muscles, tissues, etc. The brain fills the hollow of the skull, the spinal cord fills the hollow of the spine, and many nerves are filling spaces in the body. The nerve tissue also functions as the main communication system in our bodies, connecting everything to everything else (like Wi-Fi). These deep, powerful, and all-permeating channels are very important (aren't all the tissues?). Without marrow, our body does not regenerate; no new cells are created. And without the nervous system, nothing happens. I often describe the nervous system as the part of our biology that monitors, oversees, and integrates all the other systems.

As someone who had seizures for a decade, I have a unique relationship with my nervous system. I have learned to gauge when it's on high alert, overdrive, and even depletion. Any of these imbalances made it more likely that I would have a seizure. Again, balance of healthy tissues is key.

Recommendations for Marrow and Nervous System

1. Consume bone broth.

We learned earlier that like increases like, so if we want to build bone tissue, then we benefit from consuming bone tissue. One of the most accessible forms is bone broth. When I have time, I make my own (I use the slow cooker function of my Instant Pot to cook it overnight), which is the ideal. However, when I don't have time to make my own, I buy organic chicken broth that doesn't have a bunch of extra additives that I can't pronounce. I have a rule that if I can't pronounce the word, I don't put it in my body—and I practice the Sanskrit language, so that says something.

2. Eat healthy fats.

Ayurveda's golden child is *ghee*, which is clarified butter. This is a wonderfully nourishing healthy fat for the nerve tissue. I have also used high-quality fish oil (some fish oils have the healthy fats, and some have scary chemicals too, so please read the labels!) with great success. Ayurveda also recommends warm spiced organic whole milk; warm means the milk is heated (not cold milk, which is very hard to digest), and spiced means it's mixed with some turmeric, cinnamon, ginger, and honey. Bone marrow is also a great fat. The way I get this one is by adding 1 teaspoon of apple cider vinegar when I make bone broth, and this pulls the marrow out of the bones and into the broth. Sesame oil also gets honourable mention and is considered "nourishing for all the tissues." Nuts and seeds are also high in healthy fats that support the nourishment of brain tissue: in particular pumpkin seeds, almonds, and walnuts.

3. Eat dark chocolate.

If you know me well, you are already smiling. As I was looking up foods that support each tissue, dark chocolate was listed as a food that supports the nerve tissue due to its flavanol content. Best. Day. Ever. 🖤

There is a catch, though. The higher the cacao content, the more flavanols are present. A chocolate that is 70% or higher in its cacao content is recommended. Also consider how many additional ingredients there are—the fewer the ingredients, the better, as this makes it easier to digest. Milk chocolate and white chocolate do not have this benefit.

Remember that there comes a point with the consumption of any substance (including dark chocolate) where the amount changes the effects in our body. Quantity can turn a medicine to a poison. I wrote this reminder as much for myself as for you. Overdosing on chocolate reduces the health benefits. Ayurveda is about finding balance in your system.

4. Calm your nervous system.

This recommendation supports nervous function more than the marrow itself. When the marrow decreases and the nervous function is impaired, it is important to stabilize the nervous system, given that it regulates so many other systems and functions.

Being in stress mode, known as "fight or flight," causes a cascade of hormones and neurotransmitters to be released into the body. These are hard on the tissues. They are degenerative, which means they break things down. If we are in this stress mode frequently, it causes a breakdown of our tissues and impairs various functions in the body. When under stress, some people get digestive issues (this means *agni* goes offline!), other people get headaches, others get rashes, and some people get emotional (whether it's angry, anxious, or depressed). Whatever that looks like for you, it's not a sign of health—it's a sign that something is out of balance.

Figuring out what you need to do to move out of fight or flight (sympathetic branch of your autonomic nervous system) into rest and digest (parasympathetic branch of your autonomic nervous system) is important for the health of the nerve tissue, and all your other tissues too. Some people calm down by listening to music, doing yoga (which includes movement, breathing, meditation, chanting, etc.), taking time outside in nature, or spending time with good friends. Whatever your recipe for calm, schedule it in regularly so your nerves can settle and your system can relax.

A very popular option with my clients is Yoga Nidra meditation. It's one of my favourites too. Yoga Nidra meditation is a type of meditation where you are guided through the whole meditation. One bonus is that you can practice it lying down, which people sometimes prefer to seated meditations. It is very grounding, and for a lot of people it's deeply relaxing. It is a great way to calm the mind, nerves, and entire system.

Seventh Tissue—Reproductive (*Shukra*)

The seventh tissue is reproductive tissue. This is sperm for men and ova for women. The function of reproductive tissue is survival of the species, the ability to reproduce, and it contains within it the essence of all tissues via the DNA it shares.

The male *shukra* is the sperm. Sperm is produced by the testicles and moves through the epididymis to the seminal vesicle for maturation. When it's time for release, the sperm moves through the urethra and out of the body. These are the male channels of reproduction. Making sure these channels are clear and that the sperm is healthy are important signs of health for men. If the channels are blocked, or the sperm is weak, this is a sign of imbalance.

The female *shukra* is the ovum, which is released from the ovaries into the fallopian tubes. The fallopian tubes guide the ovum into the uterus. If there is sperm present to fertilize the egg, the fertilized egg can implant and mature in the uterus. If no fertilization occurs, the ovum turns into menstrual fluid (called *artava* in Sanskrit) and moves out of the uterus through the vaginal opening, along with the uterine lining. The ovaries, fallopian tubes, uterus, and vagina are the female reproductive channels. The process of shedding unfertilized ovum and uterine lining is known as menstruation. For women of menstruating age, menstruation is a process that happens monthly.

Something important to mention here is that menstruation is a sign of health for women of menstruating age. A regular menstruation allows the body to move toxins and wastes out on a regular cycle, which eases the load on the lymphatic system and other channels of elimination. Not having a regular menstrual cycle is one way the body is trying to communicate with you that something is amiss. Sadly, in the modern day we have lost respect for this powerful symbol of feminine strength and health. It is referred to as the "curse" and "Aunt Flo," and we do all sorts of things to try to get rid of something we perceive as an inconvenience.

Our menstrual cycle is a sign and symbol of health. It gives us information every month on how our channels are doing, if we are maintaining balance in our system. (Guess what PMS is really about? It's a sign that your system is out of balance!) And for those who want to have children, you need to work with this channel system, not fight against it.

In the West, we are a culture that is depleted and undernourished, and one of the side effects of this is reproductive complications—whether the inability to get pregnant or stay pregnant. I am genuinely sorry if this hits a sore spot for anyone; that's not my intention. I too have lost pregnancies. I was a depleted and undernourished person until Ayurveda helped me to better nourish my tissues, right to the end of the line of tissues.

Recommendations for Reproductive Tissue

1. Consume sweet nourishing foods.

Ghee, whole milk (warmed with spices), and nuts (especially almonds) are among the best foods to support healthy reproductive tissue.

Note: Ayurvedic sweet does not refer to candy or desserts.

2. Maintain a daily routine.

A quality we want in our reproductive tissue is stability so that the tissue is able to attain full maturity. Without stability, maturity won't happen. One of the ways we increase the stable quality in Ayurveda is through daily routine, which stabilizes not only the body and digestive fire, but also the mind. This means a set wake time and bedtime, and consistent meal times. This topic is covered in more detail in Section IV of this book.

Bonus Tissue—Vital Protective Essence (*Ojas*)

Once all the tissues have been built, if there is nourishment left, *ojas* is produced.

Ojas is the vital protective essence and is related to vitality and immunity. It is the glue that cements the elements of the body together to create stability in body and mind. It circulates via the heart and throughout the body to maintain the natural resistance of all the tissues. *Ojas* production and maintenance is related to the proper functioning of the endocrine (glands and hormones), nervous, skeletal, muscular, hematopoietic (blood), and digestive systems. When all these systems perform their functions optimally, *ojas* is maintained. When a system's function goes offline (in Ayurveda we would say "becomes deranged"), our body uses this protective essence to buffer against the effects of this derangement, and any other stress.

I think of *ojas* as my resilience factor, and my buffer against the stress of life. You know how people are always talking about their well of energy? I believe *ojas* is the Sanskrit word for the well itself. And it's not just about putting energy in the well, it's about making sure the well itself is strong and stable enough to hold our vital energy (*prana*)—that our well isn't cracked or leaking. When my well of *ojas* is low, it feels like everything is the "straw that breaks the camel's back." When I have plenty of *ojas*, I can handle a lot of challenges with grace and ease.

The way I see it, the pillar of nourishment is all about building *ojas*—this protective container that holds our energy and buffers our system against the damaging effects of stress. If we have quality nourishment, the digestive strength to digest it, and the ability to convert it into healthy strong tissues, we also build *ojas* to keep us resilient and healthy.

How do I maintain my ojas?

This is a fabulous and important question. The first thing to look at is what depletes your *ojas*:

Stress

Stress requires a lot of resources and energy from us. Being under a lot of stress, or a medium amount of stress a lot of the time, means that we are using *ojas* all the time to buffer the harmful effects of stress on our biology. The more stress we are under, the more *ojas* we use up.

Trauma

Another way to describe trauma is as a huge stressor. It might be a one-time deal, or it might go on for years. Either way, the more intense the trauma, or the more trauma you experience, the more *ojas* your biology uses to buffer the harmful effects of the stress response on your system.

Lack of Nourishment

Since *ojas* is a product of digestion, and it is the last tissue built from what we consume as nourishment, if we do not have enough nourishment, we won't be able to produce *ojas*.

Improper Eating

This can include not eating enough food (like the previous point), though it also includes eating the foods that you can't digest or are sensitive or allergic to. Kale may be a "healthy," nutrient-dense vegetable, yet if your *agni* cannot break it down in order to absorb the nutrients, it is not healthy for you.

Improper Lifestyle

This refers to day-to-day choices in your lifestyle that create stress on your system. It can be anything from staying up too late, skipping meals, not getting enough sleep, the stress of feeling rushed and overscheduled, or not exercising enough. It refers to any daily choices that are not moving you in the direction of your health, or that are moving you in the direction of stress.

Excess on Any Level

This is too much of anything: too much food, too much sleep, too much sex (remember, *ojas* is produced after the reproductive tissues; too much sex = not enough nutrition for *ojas*), working too hard, stressing too much, burning the candle at both ends, overusing your sense organs (too much TV, smells, tastes, sounds, touch, etc.), processing or experiencing a lot of emotional energy (emotions, feelings), and overthinking. As soon as you do something past your body-mind's ability to tolerate it, you start using your *ojas* to buffer the effects.

Holding onto Emotions

Of the emotional energies, there are three that use a lot of *ojas* to buffer our systems against their strength: anger, grief, and worry. In my experience of these emotions, they are strong, they can take over, they are difficult to process (or we could say "digest"), and so they churn. It is the churning, stewing, chewing, "hamster running in the wheel"-ness of these emotions that make them more *ojas* depleting.

Before we get anti-emotion (please don't go that route), know that there are emotions that also build *ojas*, like joy, love, and contentment. It's not about "not feeling," it's about finding healthy ways to work with our emotions so they don't consume us and eat up all our *ojas*.

Hunger and Thirst

Hunger and thirst are signs that nourishment is required. This is an important awareness for individuals who choose to fast (which is abstaining from food and/or drink to varying degrees). Stay mindful of the point in the fast where you aren't clearing your channels anymore; you're simply using up *ojas*.

Another situation where hunger and thirst can happen is if someone is living in poverty. There are a lot of factors in this context that are *ojas* depleting.

Relationships

This is an interesting one. Relationships can either build or deplete your *ojas*. A relationship that is supportive, growth-promoting, and loving builds your *ojas* (and theirs). A relationship that is stressful or abusive depletes your *ojas*.

How do I build ojas?

The three pillars of health, the ones I am sharing with you in this book, are how we build our *ojas*. There are specifics in terms of diet and lifestyle. Let's look at these:

Ojas-Building Foods

Ojas-building foods are nutrient dense and tissue building. These include:

- Fresh, local, seasonal foods—things grown close to home are the best medicine for us
- Organic *ghee* and warm spiced organic milk
- Kitchari—this is a blend of white basmati rice, yellow split mung beans, and digestive spices
- Molasses and maple syrup
- Almonds
- Sweet potatoes
- Sweet fruits—like berries, dates, grapes, and raisins
- Organic bone broth and organic meats
- Food prepared with love—love builds *ojas* ♥

Remember, if you cannot digest it, it does not build your *ojas*.

Ojas-*Building Lifestyle*

We can use our lifestyle, which is how we live our lives day to day, to either build our *ojas* or deplete it. The following life-style elements are considered *ojas*-building:

1. Take breaks and rest.

This includes:

- **Restorative sleep:** See pillar 2.

- **Energy management:** See pillar 3.

- **Daily routine:** A consistent daily routine creates a stable rhythm, which strengthens the body and helps to make it more efficient.

- **Retreat:** Taking a break from your regular routine can refresh the body, mind, and heart. This might be going to a cottage, camping, taking a day trip, practicing yoga, or undertaking a meditation retreat. There are so many retreat options.

- **Time in nature:** Mother Nature is naturally *ojas*-building. Maybe this is nature gazing or walking in a park or con-servation area. Spending time outside not only calms the nervous system (less stimulation), it also nourishes the senses, calms the mind, and builds *ojas*.

- **Media fasting:** Take a break from screens and technol-ogy to let your nervous system calm down and move from sympathetic (fight or flight) into parasympathetic (rest and digest).

2. Prioritize self-care.

- **Reduce stress:** Stress is a huge *ojas*-depleting factor, so consider any current stressors that you can eliminate: work, home, relationships, life, family, too much stuff, too many things to do.

- **Daily oil self-massage:** This is the same practice we discussed to care for the skin. It also provides nourishment to the tissues from the outside in, as well as calming the nervous system.

- **Yoga:** Yoga can be a fabulous *ojas*-building practice. That said, not all yoga builds *ojas*—some approaches to practice are depleting, and if you're depleted, what you're depleting is your *ojas*. The styles of practice that are very *ojas*-building include gentle, restorative, yin, and yoga therapy. *Mantra* and meditation also build *ojas*. Some of the breath work builds *ojas*, like alternate nostril breathing, mindful breathing, and the bumblebee breath. Practicing in community where you are connecting to others in an inspired way builds *ojas*, as do kirtan and prayer.

- **Mindful eating:** Focusing on your food, slowing down to eat, chewing your food, tasting your food, savouring your food, enjoying your meal. These build *ojas* and support *agni*.

- **Work with your emotions:** In the West, emotions get a bad reputation, and yet they are not a bad thing—far from it! It is important to learn to work with our emotions skilfully so they don't take over our lives and deplete our *ojas*. I have a great psychotherapist who gives me useful tools to work with my emotional energy so it builds my *ojas* instead of depleting it. Journaling is one example of a tool my therapist recommends. Some folks love to journal. I am not one of those folks. That said, I appreciate that this is a great tool to get the emotional energy flowing so it doesn't clog the pipes.

- **Aromatherapy:** This is a tool used to calm the nervous system. I am not a certified aromatherapist, so I can't get into specifics. However, if this is something that interests you in terms of enhancing relaxation to build your *ojas*, reach out to a certified aromatherapist for advice.

- **Cultivate joy:** What makes you happy? Do it. Who makes you happy? Spend time with them. Being joyful and enjoying something builds *ojas*.

- **Seek out beauty:** People, places, and things that are joyful to the eyes (beauty) engage our senses in a positive way and build our *ojas*.

3. Enjoy good company.

- **Animal cuddles:** I'm not sure this would fly with classical Ayurveda, as animals were viewed differently six thousand years ago. However, I feel that modern-day animals, especially pets, are more part of the family. In this context, spending time with an animal who is giving you unconditional love is definitely *ojas*-building. I know snuggling with my puppy and kitten calms my nerves and boosts my feel-good quotient.

- **Good work:** This includes being of service to others, doing good deeds, and working in a way that is purposeful and in alignment with your purpose. This type of work is satisfying and promotes connection, community, goodwill, and satisfaction.

- **Good company:** Spend time with people who are inspiring, uplifting, supportive, loving, growth-centric, honest, and kind. These are our soul friends,[49] and soul friends build our *ojas*.

- **Sweet words:** You can compliment someone else, yourself, or receive a compliment from someone else—all of these build *ojas*. Connecting to one another from a place of love is *ojas*-building.

- **Hugs:** This is one of my favourite ways of building *ojas*! Hugs are a way of connecting lovingly with another being, and this sense of connection, acceptance, and love builds *ojas*.

- **Laughter:** This is another one of my favourites! A real belly laugh that gets energy flowing and the heart softening and opening is fabulous for building and maintaining *ojas*.

- **Love:** Loving ourselves builds our *ojas*. Loving each other builds *ojas* for both people. The vital protective energy lives in the heart and circulates via the heart. Anything that soothes and supports heart strength builds *ojas*.

---

49 This term comes from a book written by Stephen Cope of the same title. Great book.

Recommendations for *Ojas*

1. Go through the list of depleting factors and eliminate what you can.

There are some things about our lives we can change, and others we cannot. Stepping in the direction of health means looking at the things that are depleting us (a.k.a. depleting our *ojas*!) and, if it's an option, getting rid of them! Sometimes this step seems challenging; however, once you discover the benefit of having more resilience, strength, stability, and immunity, you'll wonder why you ever did those things in the first place.

2. Cultivate an ojas-rich diet and lifestyle.

Go through the lists of *ojas*-building foods and lifestyle and notice what you are already doing that builds your *ojas*. Take a moment to congratulate yourself on your healthy choices. Yay! And make sure to keep these in your day-to-day life. Now when you do these, do them with a little more attention and awareness to build even more *ojas*.

3. Consume MORE ojas-building foods and practice ojas-building lifestyle choices.

You've gone through the lists to see what you are already doing (yay you for choosing health!). Now pick something new to add to your list of *ojas*-building practices. Try one thing at a time and see how it goes for you. *Remember, building ojas can take up to 40 days, so do the practice for six weeks.* If it works for you, keep it. If it doesn't, let it go. Either way, try another, and another, and another until your well is so full and strong and your channels are so strong and clear that things flow with ease, grace, and joy.

Conclusion to the Building of Tissues

If you're here on earth, you have a body, and this body of yours is made up of tissues. The quality and quantity of these tissues largely determines how you feel in your body and how healthy you are. If your tissues are strong and healthy and are found in the right places in the proper amounts, there is a good chance you will go through life without thinking much about your tissues. What a blessing. The strength and resilience of the tissues, the amount of *ojas* you have, is a large part of this first pillar of health. On the other hand, if your tissues are not balanced, if there's too much or too little tissue, or the quality is poor, this will be an ongoing distraction and cause of suffering.

We cannot control everything. However, we can take steps to build healthier tissues and a stronger and more resilient body, which both reduces our suffering and increases our health. It's very cool.

CHAPTER 7

ELIMINATION OF BODILY WASTES

The nourishment we ingest and digest becomes our tissues. That said, not everything becomes tissue. During the process of digestion, our *agni* takes the nutrients and absorbs them and separates out the wastes for elimination. In Sanskrit, these waste products are called *malas*.

The regular elimination of these waste products is incredibly important to health. If these do not move out of the body, they clog the channels. You could think of the waste channels as part of the drains in your system. We want the drains to drain, or everything in the system backs up. In this case, the drains are made up of hollow organs that fill with waste product until full, and then the wastes need moving out. Think about what would happen if the wastes didn't move out, if the drains didn't drain. Then the entire system would back up, and the input channels would no longer be able to take things in. If this happens, no nourishment and tissue building is able to occur. All that to say, the regular elimination of our waste products is part of maintaining a healthy flow through our channel system.

The *malas* actually perform a supportive function while they're in the body. Urine and feces fill the hollow spaces of the bladder and colon, respectively, creating support and stability in those organs. Hollow organs can collapse (known as prolapse) if they are always hollow and if the tissues of the hollow organs are weak or of poor quality. This collapse, or prolapse, causes challenges to our health.

As with everything in Ayurveda, we are looking for balance. It's not just about eliminating the wastes from our channels; it's about the proper amount of waste and elimination at the proper times. If every time a few drops of urine accumulated in the bladder or some feces built up in the colon you had to go to the restroom, well, nothing else would get done. These hollow organs hold the waste products until they are "ripe," which means ready for elimination. This holding function is important too.

In my Ayurvedic practice, I talk a lot about bodily functions, including the waste products our bodies eliminate. Some people get scrunchy faced, until they understand why these wastes are important and how to read the messages our waste products share with us. Then everyone wants to talk about poop! Which is very cool, by the way.

Ayurveda describes three main waste products that are excreted from the body: feces, urine, and sweat. The idea is that if you are eating and drinking every day, then you need to be pooping, peeing, and sweating every day. Having regular bowel movements, urinating, and sweating are all SIGNS OF HEALTH. When these are excessive, reduced, or nonexistent, it's your body's way of telling you that something is up and that you need to pay attention or make a change. Let's explore each waste product and its channel of elimination, one at a time.

Feces

Since we've talked so much about digestion, let's start by talking about the waste associated directly with our digestive tract: feces, known as *purisha* in Sanskrit. After all the nutrition from our food is absorbed in our small intestine, the remnants move through the large intestine, also known as the colon. This is where it accumulates until it is ready for elimination. While the feces is in the large intestine, any excess water is absorbed. The bacteria in the colon also produce vitamins K, B1 (thiamine), and B2 (riboflavin), and they are absorbed from the colon into the bloodstream. What is not reabsorbed becomes known as feces and is eliminated from the body via the anus. This is the channel of fecal elimination. The gastrointestinal tract is food ingestion, digestion, and absorption at the top, and elimination at the bottom. Neat, eh? How interesting that this single channel performs distinct functions and gives us so much information on our state of health.

The quantity and qualities of our bowel movements tell us a lot about what's going on in our digestion:

- Consistency of the feces—watery, soft, hard, solid, semi-shaped
- Colour
- Size, amount, and shape
- Presence of undigested food in the feces
- Mucous in or on the feces
- Presence of blood
- Smell
- Does the passing of feces include pain, gas, or discomfort?

- Does the bowel movement feel complete, or does it feel like there's more to come out?
- Constipation (is it dry, or does it feel like there's too much?) or diarrhea

When I chat with people about poop, these are all the things we talk about.

Here's what I'm looking for, what I help my clients with:

✓ Regular bowel movements. If you eat every day, then it's important that you poop at least once per day.

✓ Full bowel movements. Make sure that the poop is definitely moving out, and that it feels complete.

✓ Formed, solid, and brown. This is how it should look, unless there's a reason for it to be another colour, like eating beets, taking medications, or ingesting supplements.

✓ Easy pooping. There should be no forcing, strain, discomfort, or urgency.

If you are poop curious, review the Bristol Stool Chart[50] below. It shows you seven versions of poop, and you are aiming for Type 4 the majority of the time. There's going to be variation in your bowel movements based on what's going on in your life. Since the moving of the bowels is part of the "rest and digest" part of your nervous system, the more stress you are under, the funkier the bowels get. You might also notice that when you travel, your bowel habits shift. Or if you change your diet, your poop changes. All of these variations are typical and

---

50   "Bristol Stool Chart" by Luigi970p is licensed under CC-BY-SA-3.0, https://commons.wikimedia.org/wiki/File:BristolStoolChart.png.

your body's method of communicating with you about what is happening in your digestive tract.

BRISTOL STOOL CHART		
Type 1	Separate hard lumps	SEVERE CONSTIPATION
Type 2	Lumpy and sausage like	MILD CONSTIPATION
Type 3	A sausage shape with cracks in the surface	NORMAL
Type 4	Like a smooth, soft sausage or snake	NORMAL
Type 5	Soft blobs with clear-cut edges	LACKING FIBRE
Type 6	Mushy consistency with ragged edges	MILD DIARRHEA
Type 7	Liquid consistency with no solid pieces	SEVERE DIARRHEA

Next I'm going to offer some general recommendations to support having regular bowel movements, and yet this is one of the places where I think working with someone one-on-one to support your individual needs is immensely useful. Know that this book is intended to get you started. However, if you have significant bowel issues, you have to work with someone one-on-one. This book is not likely going to do it all.

Recommendations to Support Regular Bowel Movements

1. Drink enough water.

Our entire gastrointestinal tract requires adequate lubrication and hydration in order to function optimally. This means making sure you drink enough water to keep things flowing through the channels, as well as to keep the channels clear.

This is another reason why drinking pure clean water is important to your health.

If you have dry skin and mouth and tongue, dizziness, headaches, constipation, or scanty menstruation and urination (or it's missing), these are signs of dehydration, and you may need to drink more water. The guideline for drinking water is eight 250mL glasses per day. That said, in Ayurveda we know that some folks need more, and others need less. If you need help with this, find an Ayurvedic Counsellor to guide you.

There's another aspect to this recommendation, which is making sure the water you drink is actually being absorbed into your tissues. Ever drink a lot of water and you're still thirsty? It's like you pee all the fluid out and none of it soaks in? If this happens to you, it might be helpful to use **boiled water** instead of regular water, or to add one serving of **homemade healthy hydration drink** (recipes below) to your fluid intake.

Boiled Water

Each morning I fill a large pot with water. Then I put it on the stove top and turn the burner on high to bring the water to a boil. Boil the water until ¼ (25%) of the water is evaporated, then turn off the burner. Boiling the water changes its qualities—it adds more warmth and lightness to it, making the water easier for your body to absorb. Then once it cools down a little, this is the water I drink for the day. I'll even use boiled water in the kettle and warm it back up.

Homemade Healthy Hydration Drink

This hydration drink helps your body absorb the water you drink. I use it in the summertime when I'm dehydrated, or when I'm very active like at the gym. My friend Staraya McKinstry-Robinson (a wonderful Ayurvedic Practitioner in the US) shared this recipe with our class, and I have passed it forward ever since.

1. Take 3 cups of water (that's three of the eight you need daily ☺).

2. Add the juice of a lime or lemon (use lime if you run hot, use lemon if you run cold).

3. Add sea/rock salt (I do three grinds from my grinder).

4. Add 1 tablespoon of maple syrup.

5. Stir and drink.

The salt increases water absorption into the cells. The maple syrup adds nutrition to the plasma (the plasma is our sap, and maple syrup is the sap of a tree—like increases like). The citrus boosts the *agni* so it gets well digested. I take this and split the 3 cups into two water bottles—one for the morning, and one for the afternoon.

2. When the urge to have a bowel movement arises, go poop.

For the average person, the urge to defecate arises about four times per day. When the urge arises, stop whatever you are doing and go to the restroom and poop. We often suppress our natural urges, and this is a health-demoting habit. We decide that the task at hand is more important than going to the restroom. Not fulfilling this natural biological urge not only backs up the plumbing, it also tells the body we aren't listening to its messages. What happens? Well, our plumbing gets backed up, and the body stops talking to us. Both of these outcomes are undesirable.

Of course, sometimes when the urge arises, we cannot respond to it. A great example is being in rush-hour traffic when the urge to poop arises—not much you can do there. However, if you are in a building with a restroom, and your thought is, *I'm going to finish sending this email first*, or *Once this chapter is written I will go*, or *Pooping can wait, Netflix is so much more interesting*, this is not a health-promoting choice.

3. Prioritize daily exercise.

This might be a 20-minute walk, a bike ride, or a yoga class. The human body is designed to move, and it needs to move daily for a minimum of 20 minutes. Daily movement helps to get things moving through the pipes, and that includes feces.

Yoga in particular is fabulous to support bowel movements. In yoga we move the spine in a variety of ways that creates compression and release through the tube of the torso. This offers an opportunity for all sorts of flow through the pipes, including the bowels. The best movements for supporting elimination include squatting (it's basically a "poop-tastic" pose), forward folds with abdominal compression, twisting, backbends with your belly on the floor, and flows that move the whole torso, like Sun Salutations. Yoga also works with the breath in a way that promotes a lot of circulation through the channels. This helps with pooping too. If you are unfamiliar with yoga, please learn from an experienced teacher.

4. Calm your nervous system.

Another way to look at the stress response, to view "fight or flight," is to see it as a response that causes your channels to constrict, which means to tighten. When this happens, it slows the movement of all things through the channels, including feces. Excess stress can slow down our bowel movements.

Figuring out what you need to do to calm your nervous system is important for digestive health, including being able to poop.

Urine

Our blood is filtered through the kidneys to remove excess particulate and waste products. Once the kidneys filter out these products, the wastes move down the ureters (channels that connect the kidneys to the bladder) for storage in the bladder until it is time for elimination. This waste, mixed with some fluid, is known as urine, our second waste product, known as *mutra* in Sanskrit.

Most people urinate multiple times daily. This is a normal and healthy pattern. There is, of course, such a thing as too much or not enough urination.

The quantity and nature of our urine tells us a lot about what is happening in our fluid systems (blood and lymph) as well as digestion:

- Colour
- Amount
- Any particulate in the urine—including mucous, blood, or anything else
- Smell

- If urination includes pain or discomfort
- Does urination feel complete, or is it like there's more and it's not coming out?
- Inability to urinate, or inability to hold the urine in
- Is there hesitancy, urgency, or difficulty?
- Excessive urination, or urination at un-ideal times (like in the middle of the night)

When I chat with people about pee, these are all the things we talk about.

Here's what I'm looking for, what I help my clients with:

✓ Regular urination. You should feel the urge to urinate multiple times per day during the waking hours.

✓ Full urination. It feels complete.

✓ Yellow. Urine should be a light-yellow colour unless there's a reason for it to be another colour, like eating beets, taking medications, or ingesting supplements. The darker the yellow, the more water you need to drink.

✓ Easy urination. There should be no forcing, strain, discomfort, or urgency.

Recommendations to Support Healthy Urination

1. Drink enough water.

Our kidneys help to regulate the fluid balance of our cardio-vascular system. In order to urinate, there has to be enough water/fluids in the system for the kidneys to move any excess out. This means making sure you drink enough water that there is extra to urinate wastes out of your body. This is another reason why drinking pure clean water is important to your health.

If you have dry skin and mouth and tongue, dizziness, head-aches, constipation, or scanty menstruation and urination (or it's missing), these are signs of dehydration, and you may need to drink more water. The guideline for drinking water is eight 250mL glasses per day. That said, in Ayurveda we know that some folks need more, and others need less. If you need help with this, find an Ayurvedic Counsellor to guide you.

Boiled Water

Each morning I fill a large pot with water. Then I put it on the stove top and turn the burner on high to bring the water to a boil. Boil the water until ¼ (25%) of the water is evaporated, then turn off the burner. Boiling the water changes its qualities—it adds more warmth and lightness to it, making the water easier for your body to absorb. Then once it cools down a little, this is the water I drink for the day. I'll even use boiled water in the kettle and warm it back up.

Homemade Healthy Hydration Drink

This hydration drink helps your body absorb the water you drink. I use it in the summertime when I'm dehydrated, or when I'm very active like at the gym. My friend Staraya McKinstry-Robinson (a wonderful Ayurvedic Practitioner in the US) shared this recipe with our class, and I have passed it forward ever since.

1. Take 3 cups of water (that's three of the eight you need daily ☻).
2. Add the juice of a lime or lemon (use lime if you run hot, use lemon if you run cold).
3. Add sea/rock salt (I do three grinds from my grinder).
4. Add 1 tablespoon of maple syrup.
5. Stir and drink.

The salt increases water absorption into the cells. The maple syrup adds nutrition to the plasma (the plasma is our sap, and maple syrup is the sap of a tree—like increases like). The citrus boosts the *agni* so it gets well digested. I take this and split the 3 cups into two water bottles—one for the morning, and one for the afternoon.

2. When the urge to urinate arises, go pee.

For the average person, the urge to urinate arises every one to two hours during the day. When the urge arises, stop whatever you are doing and go to the restroom and pee. We often suppress our natural urges, and this is an unhealthy habit. As we discussed above, not fulfilling this natural biological urge not only backs up the plumbing, it also tells the body we aren't listening to its messages. What happens? Well, our plumbing gets backed up, and the body stops talking to us. Both these outcomes are unhelpful on the path to health.

Of course, sometimes when the urge arises, we cannot respond to it. A great example is being in rush-hour traffic when the urge to urinate arises—not much you can do there. However, if you are in a building with a restroom, and your thought is *I'm going to finish this Sun Salutation first*, or *I want to finish putting away the dishes*, or *Peeing can wait—this documentary on Ayurveda is so much more interesting*, this is not a health-promoting choice.

3. Practice a post-urination bladder squeeze.

There's a technique I learned to make sure the bladder is empty, and that urination is complete for those who sit to urinate. At the end of urination, while still sitting on the toilet, lift your heels, bring the palms of your hands to your low belly (below your belly button), and forward fold over your hands and thighs. This squeezes any remaining fluid out of the bladder.

Another health-promoting practice for women is to make sure they urinate after having sexual intercourse. This significantly reduces the likelihood of bladder infections.

Sweat

The third main channel of waste elimination is through the skin via sweat, known as *sveda* in Sanskrit. Unlike the other two main waste elimination channels, this one is external, meaning on the outside of our bodies. Our skin is the largest organ and has many important functions including protection (immunity), regulation of body temperature, carrier (what goes on the skin gets absorbed into the blood), and sensation. It protects the body from external infections like viruses, bacteria, fungi, parasites, etc. The skin helps the body to regulate its temperature via vasodilation (the channels expand so the body can release heat and doesn't overheat), vasoconstriction (the channels tighten so the body keeps the heat it has so it doesn't get too cold), and sweating. The skin has a strong connection to the nervous system, which regulates its various functions, and the skin is the sense organ that receives tactile information. Maintaining the health of the skin supports all of its functions.

When it comes to the skin, here are some of the things we want to assess:

- Tone of the skin. Is it plump and firm, or loose and saggy?
- Is your skin dry, itchy, or oozy?
- Any spots, patches, rashes, acne, or lesions?
- Are you able to sweat easily? Can you sweat at all? Do you sweat all the time? Does your sweat smell?
- Do you put anything on your skin? If yes, what?

Here's what I'm looking for, what I help my clients with:

- ✓ Healthy, hydrated skin
- ✓ Clear skin
- ✓ Able to sweat proportionately to the amount of exertion

Recommendations to Support Healthy Skin and Sweating

1. Sweat daily.

In order to eliminate waste through the skin, you have to sweat every day. You can sweat either through internal or external heat. External heat includes a hot room or sauna. The external heat opens the pores and sweat comes out, bringing toxins with it. Internal heat refers to warming the body up through movement and exercise to get the pores open and the sweat flowing.

2. Keep your agni strong.

A lot of *ama* comes out through the skin or surfaces as skin issues like pimples, acne, rashes, psoriasis, rosacea, eczema, etc. Since *ama* is a product of compromised digestion, in order to have healthy and clear skin, we have to keep our *agni* strong and our *ama* low. This includes not overeating, focusing on eating healthy foods, and eating good-quality nourishing foods.

3. Drink enough water.

Our entire gastrointestinal tract requires adequate lubrication and hydration in order to function optimally. We also need to have enough fluid in the body for the body to release water through perspiration. This means making sure you drink enough water to keep things flowing through the channels, as well as to keep the channels clear. This is another reason why drinking pure clean water is important to your health.

If you have dry skin and mouth and tongue, dizziness,

headaches, constipation, or scanty menstruation and urination (or it's missing), these are signs of dehydration, and
you may need to drink more water. The guideline for drinking
water is eight 250mL glasses per day. That said, in Ayurveda
we know that some folks need more, and others need less.
If you need help with this, find an Ayurvedic Counsellor to
guide you.

There's another aspect to this recommendation, which is
making sure the water you drink is actually being absorbed
into your tissues. Ever drink a lot of water and you're still
thirsty? It's like you pee all the fluid out and none of it soaks
in? If this happens to you, it might be helpful to use **boiled
water** instead of regular water, or to add one serving of **homemade healthy hydration drink** (recipe below) to your fluid
intake.

Boiled Water

Each morning I fill a large pot with water. Then I put it
on the stove top and turn the burner on high to bring
the water to a boil. Boil the water until ¼ (25%) of the
water is evaporated, then turn off the burner. Boiling the
water changes its qualities—it adds more warmth and
lightness to it, making the water easier for your body to
absorb. Then once it cools down a little, this is the water
I drink for the day. I'll even use boiled water in the kettle
and warm it back up.

Homemade Healthy Hydration Drink

This hydration drink helps your body absorb the water
you drink. I use it in the summertime when I'm dehydrated, or when I'm very active like at the gym. My friend

Staraya McKinstry-Robinson (a wonderful Ayurvedic Practitioner in the US) shared this recipe with our class, and I have passed it forward ever since.

1. Take 3 cups of water (that's three of the eight you need daily ☺).
2. Add the juice of a lime or lemon (use lime if you run hot, use lemon if you run cold).
3. Add sea/rock salt (I do three grinds from my grinder).
4. Add 1 tablespoon of maple syrup.
5. Stir and drink.

The salt increases water absorption into the cells. The maple syrup adds nutrition to the plasma (the plasma is our sap, and maple syrup is the sap of a tree—like increases like). The citrus boosts the *agni* so it gets well digested. I take this and split the 3 cups into two water bottles—one for the morning, and one for the afternoon.

4. Practice oil self-massage.

This is a classic Ayurveda self-care practice that provides nourishment to the tissues from the outside in, which supports the health of the skin and calms the nervous system. Since the skin is our largest organ, and an organ of waste elimination, taking good care of its tissues is very important. For this practice we use food grade oils, like sesame, coconut, sunflower, sweet almond, or *ghee* to feed the skin. It is important for *agni* to be strong in order to digest the oil coming in from the skin.

This practice is best done before showering (apply the oil, let your skin absorb it, then wash off any excess in the shower using a natural soap), or in the evening before bed where you can let the skin absorb the nutrition overnight. Excess oil has to be washed off, else it can clog the pores, which defeats the purpose.

Note: If you are having challenges with your skin (like pimples, acne, rashes, psoriasis, rosacea, etc.) you might hold off on applying oil until the skin calms down and the rashes (etc.) clear. It would be better to focus on strengthening *agni* and clearing *ama*, than applying oil to the skin.

Conclusion to the Elimination of Wastes

Just as taking in good-quality nourishment is important for health, so is moving the things the body does not need out of our system. And the feelings, thoughts, and memories we don't need out of our heart-minds too! The daily moving out of waste products helps keep the channels open and clear. After all, how do you think *ama* moves out? It gets digested by *agni*, or it moves through our feces, urine, or sweat. Didn't I mention that the body was designed brilliantly to take care of getting rid of the wastes? Now we know how, and how to better support these important channels of outflow.

CHAPTER 8

CONCLUSION TO PILLAR 1

Nourishment is the first pillar of health, and yet there is so much more to this pillar than simply eating well. We need to support our digestion so we can nourish ourselves and reduce the amount of metabolic waste we build up. The nourishment leads to building tissues and *ojas*, our resilience and immunity. Then we also have to be able to eliminate the wastes, the things that we cannot digest, in order to keep the channels open so things can flow.

There's a lot of moving pieces to this idea of health, and yet each piece can be worked on one at a time. Once one piece improves, you'll notice that many things shift. Changing either how you eat or what you eat will affect your tissues and your elimination, and that's just the beginning.

You might want to reread this section after reading about the other two pillars of health. This is the kingpin pillar, hence why it's the first. If we don't get our digestion, tissue building, and elimination sorted, health will continue to be elusive. As we strengthen our *agni*, reduce our *ama*, build healthy tissues, and eliminate our wastes—well, now we have a finely oiled machine that is purring like a kitten. Consider what steps you will take in the direction of becoming a finely oiled machine. Meow. ☺

Now that you have read this section, consider the following:

1. What are you already doing to keep your *agni* (digestive fire) strong? Remember to keep this!

2. What is one thing you could do to boost your *agni* (digestive fire)?

3. What are you already doing to reduce or remove *ama* (metabolic waste)? Remember to keep this!

4. What is one thing you could do to reduce or remove *ama* (metabolic waste)?

5. Are there any tissues you might want to focus on?

6. Is there a waste elimination that you want to focus on?

SECTION III:

PILLAR 2

SLEEP

*Sleep is the golden chain that binds
health and our bodies together.*

—Thomas Dekker

Introduction to Pillar 2

Ayurveda's second pillar of health is sleep, called *nidra* in Sanskrit.

In my experience, people understand why sleep is important. I think we've all had an experience of sleep deprivation (whether for fun reasons or not so fun), and we know that we are not at our best the next day. Our brain is slow and foggy, our body is achy and doesn't respond the same. We're shorter on patience and the ability to problem solve.

We are at our best with the appropriate amount of sleep. Let's dive right into this pillar of health!

CHAPTER 9

IMPORTANCE OF SLEEP

Why Is Sleep Important?

There is a great passage from one of Ayurveda's classical texts, the *Ashtanga Samgraha*, on sleep. Vagbhata says,

> Obesity and emaciation, happiness and sorrow, strength and weakness, virility and impotence, knowledge and ignorance, life and death, are all dependent on adequate and inadequate sleep.

> Sleep indulged into at improper time, in excess or not at all, destroys one's happiness and life just as the black night just prior to death.

> The same sleep indulged into judiciously will make for happiness and long life just as the mind of the yogis become clear from the knowledge of the soul and penances.[51]

So if we want to have healthy tissues, maintain balance in the body and mind, and cultivate happiness, strength, virility, knowledge, and longevity, adequate sleep is crucial.

---

51 From the *Ashtanga Samgraha, Sutrasthana 9.22–9.24*.

What Does Sleep Do?

There is a lot of information and research that exists around what sleep does. Restorative sleep provides us with many benefits in all our dimensions of being—the body, energy, emotions, mind, and spirit.

The benefits of sleep include:

- Natural detoxification of tissues: *agni* is working to clear the *ama* from our tissues and channels, moving the wastes to our gastrointestinal tract for elimination

- Cellular restoration: our cells take the time to rebuild, nourish, and strengthen

- Emotional processing: an opportunity to digest and integrate our emotions, as well as move any emotional *ama* out

- Enhanced memory and retention: also an opportunity to digest our thoughts and experiences

- Rest for the sense organs and nervous system: by releasing our connection to the stimulation of the world, the senses (and nervous system, which processes the sensory data) get a break, which reduces the tendency to overuse our sense organs

- Allostatic load is resolved, which means allowing the body to go back to its normal state after being in the stress response, a time to shift from the sympathetic into the parasympathetic.

Sleep is restorative for the body and mind. It relieves stress by slowing down the heart and breathing rates, which reduces our oxygen requirements.

Restorative sleep is a sign of healthy, natural biological rhythms. When we aren't sleeping well, it's a sign that something is off balance, and we need to course correct. There are a ton of reasons why our sleep can become disturbed, including late nights (missing the ideal window to fall asleep), stress, illness, grief, worry, being overly busy, disturbance (like loud neighbours, young children, and pets!), and having too much of the light quality since we need a certain amount of heaviness to fall asleep.

How Much Sleep Do I Need?

It depends. Different people need different amounts of sleep. Some people function well with six hours, whereas others need eight or nine hours of sleep. Through exploration and contemplation, you'll figure out the amount of sleep you need. Also, if you're sick, stressed, or have a heavy emotional load, you'll need more sleep. If you're doing a lot of meditation practice, you might function well with less sleep.

Here's another great place for a reminder that what we are looking for is balance. If you don't get enough sleep, your function and sense of well-being are compromised. AND if you get too much sleep, your function and sense of well-being are also compromised. Interesting how the dosage matters, even in sleeping. Remember to think Goldilocks—not too much, not too little, just right! And just right for you might be different than for someone else. Part of this exploration is to figure that out.

For example, I know that I need eight hours of sleep a night to function optimally. By function optimally, I mean that my body feels strong, I have the energy to get through my day, my emotions are not leaking out of me, my mind is online and working well, and I feel generally good moving through my life. If I oversleep, I notice right away that my body feels heavier and my mind is more cloudy and dull. If I don't sleep enough, my body feels agitated and my mind is jumpy and all over the place.

Why Is It the Second Pillar?

Ever wonder why sleep isn't Ayurveda's first pillar of health? I know some folks believe in random chance, yet Ayurveda is not random at all. Everything is really well thought out, and everything is in the order it's in for a reason.

It turns out that your body needs fuel to make the transition from waking state to sleep state. If your tank is empty, you can't fall asleep. Have you ever been super exhausted and yet unable to fall asleep? Empty tank = no sleep.

This is why the sleep pillar follows the nourishment pillar. Once the body is well nourished, it has the resources to shift gears from awake to asleep.

Recommendations to Support Restorative Sleep

Many people suffer from sleep disturbances, including insomnia. This is something I see a lot in my Ayurvedic practice. I'm happy to say that Ayurveda has a lot of recommendations to support getting better and deeper sleep. Try them to see if they support you in getting a good night's sleep on a regular basis!

1. Maintain a consistent bedtime.

Having a consistent bedtime (and wake time too) is a great way to get the body and mind into a stable rhythm that supports deep restorative sleep. When our bedtime is variable, which means always changing, the body doesn't know when to wake up or stay asleep. When you bring consistency to your bedtime and wake time, your body knows when to wind down and settle in for rest. Sometimes we need to retrain healthy habits into the body, especially if it has fallen out of sync.

Ayurveda recommends that most people go to bed around 9:30 p.m. and aim to be asleep around 10 or 10:30 p.m. This is in line with modern research around sleep hormones (see the section about melatonin below). A lot of folks get a second wind between 10 and 11 p.m., and if you're not settled and sleeping before that second wind, the next thing you know it is 1:30 a.m. and you missed your sleep window. Being awake between 11 p.m. and 2 a.m., which is when your body does its self-cleaning, is a missed opportunity for your body to naturally detoxify while you rest. If this goes on for a prolonged amount of time, *ama* builds up, and the door to imbalance and disease opens.

The other piece to the "going to bed on time" puzzle is making sure that you are getting up at a consistent time. Ayurveda recommends getting up before the sun. A good guideline is between 5:30 and 6 a.m. When we get up early, we tend to get tired around 9:30 p.m. Those who sleep until 7 or 8 a.m. wake up with a foggy brain and fluctuating energy throughout the day. My clients who commit to early rising (before 6 a.m.) and early bedtime (by 9:30 p.m.) report having more energy, stable energy, fewer food cravings, and better sleep. I found this to be true for me too.

2. Keep your bedroom dark for sleep.

The body has certain functions that are triggered by light and dark. How amazing is that?! When it's light out (daytime), the body produces more cortisol, one of the hormones that activates and stimulates the body (cortisol is a primary sympathetic nervous system hormone). When it's dark out (nighttime), the body reduces its cortisol production and increases the production of melatonin, which invites the body to move from alertness to sleepiness.

Understanding this important play of hormones and taking steps to have a dark bedroom supports deep and restorative sleep. Replace screens (like TVs) and bright lights with softer lighting, and use shades over windows, or use an eye mask.

3. Only use your bedroom for sleep and sex.

If we want our sleep to be deep and restful, then we want to create a peaceful and relaxing environment in the room itself. If you use your bedroom for work or entertainment (like watching movies), then when you go to bed, thoughts related to these activities might come up. If the bedroom is only for sleep and sex, then being in your bedroom will likely bring up thoughts of sleep or sex.

4. Minimize screen time before bed.

Turns out that screens (this is all technology, from cell phones to monitors to TVs) are very stimulating for the nervous system. When the nervous system is stimulated, cortisol is released, which we know stimulates and awakens the mind. Going screen-free one or two hours before bed can be immensely helpful. Instead try reading, journaling, doing gentle yoga, or listening to a guided meditation.

5. Finish dinner two hours before bed.

Eating too close to bedtime means the body is digesting instead of resting. A big meal or heavy foods require a very strong *agni* and are more likely to produce *ama* when consumed in the late evening. If you go to bed with a full tummy, then instead of your body cleansing itself between 11 p.m. and 2 a.m., it spends that energy digesting the food. This can lead to poor sleep and weight gain as *ama* accumulates.

6. Avoid stimulants and stimulation before bed.

Stimulants, such as alcohol, activate the nervous system instead of calming it down for rest. Many people think that alcohol relaxes them, and the routine of having a glass of wine in the evening might do just that. However, alcohol is a stimulant to the system until the body can no longer digest the alcohol, then it becomes a depressant.

A variety of stimulants have the same pattern as alcohol. If it's the unwinding routine that benefits you, try it with something else like your favourite tea.

Stimulation includes screens (mentioned above), checking email, exercise, stressful/emotional/intense conversations, or anything that will overly engage the senses.

7. Enjoy a cup of herbal tea or warm spiced milk.

Wives tales, yes. Effective, also yes. A cup of warming herbal tea, like chamomile or tulsi, can relax the nerves, which prepares you for sleep. A cup of warm spiced milk (whatever milk you drink—cow, sheep, almond, cashew, or hemp) also works very well. The spices I most enjoy in my spiced milk are ground ginger, turmeric, and cinnamon with a touch of honey to sweeten it. Feeling warm and cozy on the inside will help the body-mind settle into rest.

8. Give yourself a foot massage with warm oil.

This is a very traditional Ayurvedic recommendation. The types of oil that are really good for this include sesame, sweet almond, mustard seed, jojoba, or coconut (coconut for the summer and for sensitive skin). Please do not put anything on your skin that you are allergic to or that you would not eat. Take a bit of oil in your hands and rub it between the palms to warm the oil. Mindfully massage the oil into your feet.

The feet have many *marma* (acupressure) points, as well as fascial connections throughout the body. As you massage your feet, your whole body relaxes, and when this happens, so does your mind. It is a wonderfully grounding and nourishing self-care practice. After the foot massage, put some socks on and hop into bed for a deep and relaxing sleep.

Sometimes my husband and I will massage each other's feet before bed, which is lovely for both of us. I know not everyone likes having his or her feet touched. If you do, try this recommendation.

9. Establish a pre-bedtime routine.

We've talked already about how routines are stabilizing for the body and grounding for the mind. Establishing a "pre-bedtime" routine can be powerful for training the body-mind to get ready for sleep.

Mine includes things like walking the dog, having a cup of warm water, putting away the dishes and turning on the dishwasher, brushing and flossing my teeth, putting out my clothes for the next day, writing down any lingering mental to-dos, then doing a Sudoku with my hubby before falling asleep.

I have many clients who practice gentle yoga, meditate, journal, listen to relaxing music, or take a warm bath. You can include any of the items on this list, or things that you know help you sleep at night. Everyone's bedtime routine will need to be unique to them.

10. Try a Yoga Nidra meditation.

With clients who have long-standing insomnia, I recommend they listen to a Yoga Nidra meditation before bed. Many fall asleep during this type of guided meditation because it can be so relaxing. Although this isn't the point of the meditation, it's a side effect I see often, and when we need sleep, we have to try anything that could work. With Yoga Nidra you would set up the recording to play as you relax into bed. The idea is to follow the meditation, which brings you into deeper states of relaxation. The hope is that eventually you fall asleep.

There are many wonderful Yoga Nidra meditations. I have some for download on my website. I listen to Swami Jnaneshvara

Bharati's "Extreme Relaxation." Anything by Richard Miller PhD, Joy Kristin, or Jennifer Reis will be helpful. Keep working with them until you find the voice and meditation that works for you, then use it to rest, relax, and help you sleep.

CHAPTER 10

CONCLUSION TO PILLAR 2

My hope is that the information in this section serves you in consistently getting good sleep. We've all felt the benefits of, and know the importance of, restorative sleep. Sometimes we have to put more time and effort into making sure that we are able to sleep well, and not taking these steps is a misuse of the intellect (remember this from the causes of disease in Section I?). The more you invest in sleeping well, the more this pillar can support your health in a profound and stable way.

Now that you have read this section, consider the following:

1. What are you already doing to help you sleep well? Remember to keep this!

2. Which of the recommendations will you explore to sleep better?

SECTION IV:

PILLAR 3

ENERGY MANAGEMENT

*Balance is not something you find,
it's something you create.*

—Jana Kingsford

Introduction to Pillar 3

Ayurveda's third pillar of health is energy management, known as *brahmacharya* in Sanskrit. There are multiple translations and interpretations for the word *brahmacharya*. All are all helpful in unraveling this concept. Let's explore them to give you a broad understanding of this pillar.

Celibacy, Sex, and *Ojas*

The traditional translation of *brahmacharya* is celibacy. Yep, as in abstention from sex. Take a breath, you'll be okay. It's not for anti-sex reasons; it is for the protection of one's *ojas*. We learned in the section about the first pillar of health that *ojas* is produced *after* the reproductive tissue is developed. If we're engaging in a lot of sex, then our biology needs to replace a lot of reproductive fluids, which reduces the chance of having enough nourishment to build our *ojas*. When we're depleted, restraining from sexual activity can give us enough resources to rebuild our *ojas*, our resilience, and immunity.

In my life as a married woman, deciding ten years into my marriage to become celibate didn't work for me. Those of us who are householders (with a marriage, mortgage, jobs, children) can practice *brahmacharya* through the idea of **respectful intimacy**. This means saving our sexual energy and experiences for a partner (or partners) that we care about, where there is mutual respect and the simultaneous cultivation of intimacy and love. Orgasm does use our reproductive fluids; however, loving intimacy builds emotional *ojas*.

Moderation

A modern translation of *brahmacharya* is moderation. This is recognizing how much energy you have and using it wisely. It is through this lens that I translate the Sanskrit into *energy management*. Picture your "well of energy"; the well itself is made of *ojas*, the container. Into the well goes your energy, called *prana*. Wise usage of our energy, the ideal, is to give only from the overflow of your *prana*. This way you have enough energy for yourself, and you're not using up the well itself to give resources you don't have.

Another way of thinking about energy management is to think of it like a bank account, one that tracks your energy. Certain ways of being—thoughts, words, and actions—deposit energy into the bank, while other things make withdrawals. As long as you are withdrawing what is in the account, you're okay energy-wise. Once you move into overdraft, this means you used up all the energy and are now using your *ojas*. Eventually, overdraft can lead to bankruptcy.

This is an interesting pillar because many people give more than they have, and this leads to depletion, depression, resentment, and burnout—and none of these are good for your health.

Energy and Age

Another interesting facet is that the amount of energy we have changes over time. We tend to have more energy in our youth (0–30 years), a reasonable amount in our adulthood (30–60 years), and then less as we enter into the golden years of life

(60+). The question is, can we honour the amount of energy we actually have, instead of constantly trying to squeeze more energy out of our systems? Do we even know how much real energy we have?

Balance, Overuse, and Underuse

In thinking about the pillars (and those of you who know me know that I've thought a lot about this), I realize there are three states that go with energy usage: overuse, balance, and underuse. Isn't it funny that we keep coming back to balance, and how the pendulum can swing in either direction from there?

Overuse is using more energy than we have—going into overdraft in the bank account. Culturally, we tend to lean on stimulants to give us "fake energy" so we can do more. These include caffeine, sugar, and processed foods.

Underuse is like turning our checking account into a savings account. The challenge with this scenario is stagnation. The lack of movement creates pooling, and this is not healthy either.

Ideally, we learn how to read our energy levels and use our energy within our capacity. We balance our energy spending with saving, so there is flow, and yet we're not running on empty. In my experience, this has two important aspects. The first is healthy boundaries, which is understanding how much energy you have and respecting that. The second is learning to say no, which supports the first. If you are asked to give more than you have, you are at risk of depleting your energy (and *ojas*). In Canada we have an organization called the OLGC, the Ontario Lottery and Gaming Corporation. They have the perfect motto for health: *Know your limit, play within it.*

Contemplations around Energy Management

There are a few important considerations in the process of working with our energy:

Where are you spending energy?

Life is multidimensional, like humans are. We use energy at work, with family, in lifestyle, with play.

What gives you energy?

We know that the first two pillars of health, nourishment and sleep, give us energy by stabilizing the well and refilling it. Perhaps other things that refill your well include work, family, friendships, lifestyle, play, etc. Did you notice that the same things that use our energy can also build our energy? Whether something gives you energy or uses your energy depends on your relationship to it, or how you relate to it.

Are you spending more energy than you are making?

If yes, recognize that this is why we get sick, depleted, and depressed. Then this leads us to another question: What can you change? Sometimes we think we have to say yes to everything and everyone, and yet, that way of living is not sustainable. In reality we have to make choices. In order to say yes to something, we have to say no to something else. If we are overspending, we are not choosing health. What can you let go of? Where can you choose differently in order to honour your own energy, vitality, and health?

Is there a dimension in your life or of your being that is using too much energy, or creating an imbalance in your system?

Once you recognize that we have physical, energetic, emotional, mental, and spiritual layers of being, ask yourself, "Is one of these using up all the energy?" Can you identify in your own experience where the energy is being used up? In my experience, pain uses up a ton of my energy, as does being overly busy.

CHAPTER 11

DAILY ROUTINE

G iven that the most powerful things we do in service (or in detriment) to our health are the things we do every day, the main recommendation to support the third pillar of health is to create an appropriate (meaning health-promoting) daily routine. In Ayurveda the daily routine, known as *dinacharya* in Sanskrit, is considered very important because it is the foundation of our lifestyle and self-care. This daily routine, when thoughtfully put together, includes steps in the direction of health, which moves us away from the causative factors of disease discussed in the first section.

The Ayurvedic daily routine helps us maintain our sense organs so they function optimally. Since the senses are how we interact with the world, their maintenance allows us to experience our lives with more clarity and more reality. Having this interaction with reality, knowing what is actually happening, keeps our minds more clear, stable, and balanced. The consistency of the daily routine provides a steadiness that supports us in stabilizing our *agni* and navigating "change over time," whether this is a seasonal transition or a phase of life transition or a transition from Sunday to Monday. From the Ayurvedic view, the deep stability provided by a health-promoting daily routine helps us to stay healthy, harmonious, and clear. It also helps us to refill the well (*prana*) and do repairs to the well itself (builds *ojas*) on a daily basis. A daily self-care routine is a requirement for health.

Interestingly, modern science is filled with research on epigenetics, which is the study of how genes are expressed in our body and their effects (not gene modification). The research demonstrates that the lifestyle we follow, the day-to-day choices we make, and our cumulative lifetime choices impact the expression of our DNA. Our gene expressions are also influenced by circadian rhythms, which refers to our biological clock that wants to align with natural rhythms. Modern science supports what Ayurveda has known for thousands of years: a daily routine strongly promotes our health and well-being.

A daily routine is a very beneficial practice for those who struggle with decision fatigue—having to make so many choices every single day. Once you have your daily routine in place, it is no longer about choice. This means you use less of your energy to make little choices, giving you more energy for the rest of your day and for the more important decisions.

Sub-Routines

I think of the daily routine as four mini-routines: one for each morning, lunch, dinner, and before bed. I use each of these sub-routines as a chance to check in with myself, to see how I'm working with my energy and how my choices are working for me. Sometimes they work great, and sometimes they don't. Each of these routines is a chance to reassess and set a new path if that's what's needed. Self-care is very dynamic, and it's important that we are open to flexibility and change as the day goes on. What seems like a good idea at 7 a.m. might not be by the time you get to 3 p.m. It's absolutely okay to change your mind and your choices as more information becomes available to you.

Morning Routine

Something I like to share with my students and clients up front is that Ayurveda is morning heavy. What I mean by that is the morning routine has the most pieces to it, and therefore is the longest of the routines. Please don't get discouraged by this; know that you will figure it out, just like I did. And the routine comes together one step at a time, one thing at a time. There is a lot in the morning routine in order to set the tone of stability, clarity, and harmony for the day—it starts your day off "on the right foot." It is also important that your self-care needs are met. Ever think to yourself "I'll do that later," and then later never comes? If you choose to get your self-care done first thing, then you are good to go for the whole day.

The basic overview of the morning routine, as described in the Ayurvedic classical texts, includes the following practices:[52]

1. Wake up before the sun.

This is considered one of the most important practices for longevity—not only in the Ayurvedic tradition, but in many other traditions as well. Waking up before the sun allows you more time in your morning so you aren't rushed. It is also a quiet time of day (especially if others are still sleeping), so the mind can go through its routine in a calm *sattvic* way. We also get up early so we have time to do our self-care.

---

52   I call them practices because you practice them every day when they are part of your daily routine.

2. Ensure morning elimination of urine and feces.

Make time in the morning to urinate and defecate. Even if you don't think you have to go, take a few minutes to sit on the toilet and breathe. Sometimes constipation comes from not making the time to poop. Allowing your body to release the wastes and *ama* from the previous day is really important to creating space for the nutrition of the day.

3. Cleanse the sense organs.

We talked about these recommendations earlier in the book, and this is where they fit into the daily routine.

- Mouth: scrape your tongue, brush your teeth, gargle, rinse, hold, or swish
- Eyes: rinse your eyes with cool water
- Nose: cleanse the nostrils with a *neti* pot + water and sea salt (if appropriate) and oil your nostrils
- Ears: use a few drops of warm oil in each ear
- Skin: dry brush, self-oil massage, and take a bath/ shower

4. Drink a glass of warm water.

This hydrates the gastrointestinal tract and clears *ama* out of the system. It is most useful to do this before putting anything else in the belly.

5. Make time for exercise: walk, yoga, etc.

Ideally a movement practice happens in the morning. This gets the body moving, gets fluids and energy circulating, and clears the cobwebs of sleep from the mind.

6. Meditate, contemplate, connect inward.

The morning is a great time to set an intention for the day, to meditate, contemplate, and connect to our deepest sense of self.

7. Eat breakfast.

Make the time to nourish yourself with breakfast. Just as you cannot drive a car with an empty tank, your biology is likely to need something in the tank to give you the energy to be present and engaged in your day. Choose something warm and nourishing that gives you enough energy to get to lunch with stability and ease.

8. Move into your day.

Maybe this means heading to work, maybe moving into parenting, maybe something else or a combination of things. The morning routine is to get you set up to be at your best for the day. Go and enjoy your day!

How our day begins has a deep impact on how our entire day unfolds. Ever have a morning that was rushed or where you ran out of time, and the rest of the day takes on that feel? We do our best here to set the tone for the whole day first thing. From here, the rest of the day is not nearly as regimented.

Lunchtime Routine

The next part of the daily routine is lunchtime. We know from the section on pillar 1 that lunch is important in terms of food consumption and digestion. Include the following in a lunchtime routine:

1. Eat your largest meal at lunch while your digestive fire is strongest.

It is also important to eat enough food to get you to dinner-time, which likely means you need more than a salad if you want to make it without tons of snacking and coffee, or a blood sugar crash at 3 p.m.

2. Rest for five minutes after eating.

If you have the space and ability, lean to your left or lie down on your left side to support digestion. Lying on your left side allows the gastric juices and your food to be in the part of your stomach that does the mixing and churning. This increases the breakdown of your food and the access to the nutrients of your food. Another way of looking at it is that resting after eating allows you more time to be in the "rest and digest" part of your nervous system. Either way, it is supportive to digestion.

3. Take 100 steps.

I have studied a lot of yoga (I'm also a yoga teacher) and pretty much every wise swami whose teachings I studied recommended taking 100 steps after every meal. If you can't walk outside (I live in Canada, and there are times of the year that it is so cold my dog won't go outside, which means I won't either!), taking 100 steps inside is doable—even if it's from one room of your apartment to another. I like this one because I noticed that as I move easily (it's not speed walking or fitness), it invites gravity to draw things down and through my digestive tract. I also feel like it relaxes my abdominal organs and keeps me from getting tired or lethargic after a meal. Movement prevents stagnation, and stagnating food is not moving us in the direction of health!

Dinner Routine

Have you noticed the pattern yet? Where there's a meal, there's a routine to go with it. The dinnertime routine includes:

1. Eat a lighter dinner.

In Ayurveda we eat the biggest meal at lunch because our digestion is stronger AND we are actively working or playing after, which gives plenty of opportunity to use up the food. Dinner is different. We're slowing down and settling in. Eat enough to satisfy your hunger, but not so much that you are stuffed. One of my teachers used to explain that "supper" comes from the word "supplementary," as in, extra or additional. It's an extra meal if you need it, yet we don't all need a lot of food late at night.

2. Rest for five minutes after eating.

If you have the space and ability, lean to your left or lie down on your left side to support digestion. Lying on your left side allows the gastric juices and your food to be in the part of your stomach that does the mixing and churning. Typically we settle in and watch something on TV after dinner, so I pick the side of the couch where I can lean on my left side after supper and it works out great.

3. Take 100 steps.

Make time for 100 steps after every meal. It supports digestion (of food and thoughts) and circulation, and it settles the nerves.

4. Have two hours between dinner and bedtime.

Sleep is disrupted if your tummy is full, so do your best to have a few hours of time for digestion between dinner and bedtime.

Bedtime Routine

In the previous chapter we talked about the many things we can do to have restorative sleep. One of the most supportive things for me is having a bedtime routine. Going through the steps of my routine helps me shift gears from an active day, unwinding for sleep. The basic bedtime routine includes:

1. Set a consistent bedtime.

Go to bed early enough to get up early and still get the amount of sleep you need to be rested. You'll need to figure out how much sleep you need and count back from your wake time. We joke in our family that 9 p.m. is "Ayurvedic Midnight." In order to get up early, you must go to bed early.

2. UNPLUG by putting away your technology 30–60 minutes before bed.

Technology, including all screens, agitates the nervous system, which interrupts your sleep. Screens particularly stimulate the eyes and brain. Putting down the iPhone and turning off Netflix allows your nervous system to unwind so you can rest.

3. Practice your end-of-day sense organ care.

Brush and floss your teeth, rinse your eyes, wash your face … you know, the typical before bed self-care things. If you feel stuffy, do another round of nasal cleansing. If you feel dry, add oil to the nose, ears, skin, or wherever it is needed.

4. Take some toilet time.

Give your body another opportunity for urination and defecation before bed. The body does best with rhythm and consistency.

5. Massage your feet with warm oil.

Self-oil massage calms the nerves, nourishes the tissues, and creates a sense of unwinding. This is a great practice before bed. If you have a partner, you can massage each other's feet before bed. I have many clients who do this for their children to help them settle more easily into sleep. It is simple and effective.

6. Enjoy a cup of warm herbal tea or spiced milk.

Something warm in the tummy helps curb hunger and calms the nervous system. I love warm spiced milk as dessert.

7. Get things ready for tomorrow.

My bedtime routine also includes less formal things like turning on the dishwasher, making sure there's clean water for our pets, and laying out my clothes for the next day. I also make a list of things I want to remember for the next day—to-do list items or important appointments. Each of these steps allows me to let go of something so I can more easily settle into sleep.

What other things make sense for you to include in your bedtime routine?

Between Routines

In between the "routines," you fill your day with what you need to—work, rest, enjoying good company, and having great adventures! A lot of people worry that having a daily routine makes their lives boring. On the contrary, it gives you more energy for the things you want to work toward and show up for. Again, between the four checkpoints, you get to fill your life with everything you want.

I know when I was first presented the daily routine idea I felt overwhelmed at how much it entails. My suggestion to students and clients isn't to tackle the whole thing today—it's to choose one thing and set the intention to do that ONE practice daily for one month. After that amount of time, you will get a sense of whether the practice serves you, and if it does, keep it. If it doesn't, let it go. And then commit to adding ONE new practice to your routine. Build your routine slowly over time. Health is a process, and we move in that direction one step at a time.

Daily Routine and the Seasons

We can adjust our routines to honour the natural shifts of each season. Here are examples of what the routine looks like for each season.

Sample Daily Schedule for Spring

- 5:30 a.m.: wake up before the sun
- 5:45 a.m.: cleansing & elimination (tongue, teeth, eyes, nose, drink warm lemon water, urinate, and poop)
- 6 a.m.: exercise, yoga, breath work, meditation

- 7 a.m.: dry brush, self-oil massage with sunflower oil, then shower/bath
- 7:30 a.m.: light breakfast
- 12 noon: lunch
- 7 p.m.: dinner
- 10 p.m.: bedtime

Sample Daily Schedule for Summer

- 5 a.m.: wake up before the sun
- 5:15 a.m.: cleansing & elimination (tongue, teeth, eyes, nose, drink warm water, urinate, and poop)
- 5:30 a.m.: exercise, yoga, breath work, meditation
- 6:30 a.m.: self-oil massage with sweet almond or coconut oil, then shower/bath
- 7 a.m.: light breakfast
- 11:30 a.m.: lunch
- 6:30 p.m.: dinner
- 9:30 p.m.: bedtime

Sample Daily Schedule for Fall

- 5:30 a.m.: wake up before the sun
- 5:45 a.m.: cleansing & elimination (tongue, teeth, eyes, nose, drink warm lemon water, urinate, and poop)
- 6 a.m.: exercise, yoga, breath work, meditation
- 7 a.m.: self-oil massage with sesame or sweet almond oil, then shower/bath
- 7:30 a.m.: light breakfast

- 12 noon: lunch
- 6 p.m.: dinner
- 9:30 p.m.: bedtime

Sample Daily Schedule for Winter

- 6 a.m.: wake up before the sun
- 6:15 a.m.: cleansing & elimination (tongue, teeth, eyes, nose, drink warm lemon water, urinate, and poop)
- 6:30 a.m.: exercise, yoga, breath work, meditation
- 7:30 a.m.: self-oil massage with sesame, sunflower, or sweet almond oil, then shower/bath
- 8 a.m.: light breakfast
- 12 noon: lunch
- 6 p.m.: dinner
- 9 p.m.: bedtime

The whole thing with the daily routine (with all the Ayurvedic recommendations) is that what every person needs is going to be slightly different because we are all slightly different. These guidelines show that as the seasons change, it makes sense to follow the natural rhythms as much as possible, and this means allowing changes to your routine from season to season. Notice the basic structure is the same; however, a few of the items change (like dry brushing might be mostly a springtime thing), and some of the timing changes (more sleep in the winter, less sleep in the spring).

Seasonal Shifts to Diet, Self-Care, and Lifestyle

I've mentioned this before: maintaining our health is a moving target. Why? Because things are constantly changing, and if we aren't paying attention to these changes, we aren't going with the flow of the natural rhythms, and this is when we get sick.

Each season has its own governing qualities, as discussed in the first section in the book. Now I want to share how we might shift our routine in some subtle and some obvious ways to continue aligning with nature to balance the change in qualities that is happening all the time.

Recommendations for Spring

1. Choose a spring season balancing diet.

We may not be able to control the season change, yet we can control what we choose to eat. Here are some broad-stroke ways to approach springtime eating:

- Favour warm, dry, light foods.
- Increase the amount of pungent, bitter, and astringent foods you eat to clear up excess mucous and fluids. Bitter and astringent foods are wonderful to dry up excess moisture in the body.
- Eat a light breakfast, and if you aren't hungry, consider skipping breakfast or having something light like baked fruit and tea.
- Eat smaller/lighter meals.

- Do not eat if you feel heavy or full.
- Reduce meat consumption, as meat is a very heavy, dense, thick food.
- Wonderful teas for the springtime include cumin-coriander-fennel (known as CCF tea) or ginger-cinnamon-raw honey.

Specific spring balancing foods include:

- Meats: venison, chicken, turkey, eggs
- Grains (light and drying): basmati rice, amaranth, barley, buckwheat, corn, millet, oats, quinoa, rye
- Legumes: split peas, red lentils, chickpeas, pinto beans, soybeans
- Fruits: apples, apricots, berries, cherries, dark grapes, peaches, pears, pomegranates, and dried fruits—this is the time of year where dried fruits can be appropriate
- Veggies: artichokes, asparagus, beets, broccoli, carrots, lettuce, okra, radish, spinach, leafy greens

2. Focus on important self-care routines for spring.

As each season has different qualities, certain self-care routines are more useful at specific times of year. Here are the ones that are most useful to bring balance to your system in the springtime:

- Exercise and sweat daily
- Gargling with salt and turmeric water
- Tongue scraping

- Nasal cleansing with a *neti* pot (unless we have too much heavy, oily, slimy/sticky, cold, and liquid qualities)
- Oil the nostrils
- Dry brushing
- Self-massage with warm sunflower oil (unless we are already oily)
- Yoga: learn some flowing sequences and warming lightening breath work from a skilled yoga teacher
- Meditation, like *kirtan* (group chanting) and walking meditation

3. Cultivate a lifestyle that balances the qualities of spring.

During the springtime, the following guidelines support balance and health:

- Stay dry.
- Choose active exercise daily. If you like more intense workouts like CrossFit or Boot Camp, this is the season for it!
- Sweat every day to melt any buildup of *ama* and mucous.
- Go outside every day and enjoy the blooming season—it lifts the spirit!
- Seek out new things—people, places, and experiences.
- Set goals and go for it!
- Spend time with friends and family.

4. Know what to reduce in the spring.

Just as there are things for us to add for each season, there are also practices to let go of. My teacher Dr. Claudia calls this "the medicine of subtraction." Sometimes, not doing something is the healthy choice.

In the spring, avoid the following:

- Raw, cold, dry, rough foods
- Heavy, oily, fried, fatty foods
- Excessive sweet, sour, salty foods
- Eating large meals
- Snacking between meals
- Cold or iced drinks
- Napping
- Complete inactivity
- Exposure to dirt, dust, and pollen
- Exposure to cold drafts from A/C

Recommendations for Summer

1. Choose a summer season balancing diet.

Here is how Ayurveda approaches summer eating:

- Favour light, cooling, and easy-to-digest foods.
- Increase the amount of sweet, bitter, and astringent foods you eat. And please remember that sweet does not mean candies and desserts. It means fruit and sweeter veggies like carrots and sweet potatoes.

- Make sure to eat breakfast to keep from getting agitated and fiery by 10 a.m.
- Reduce the consumption of red meats, as they are heating.
- *Ghee*, coconut oil, and olive oil are cooling healthy fats.
- Choose mint, nettle, or cumin-coriander-fennel (CCF) tea.

Specific summer balancing foods include:

- Meats: chicken or turkey
- Grains: basmati rice, barley, oats, wheat
- Legumes: red lentils, mung beans
- Fruits: apples, pears, melons, dates, plums, prunes, mangos
- Veggies: cucumber, lettuce, sprouts, asparagus, broccoli, sweet potatoes, salads

2. Focus on important self-care routines for summer.

Here are the most useful routines for balancing your system in the summertime:

- Exercise gently, avoid overexertion; swimming is ideal
- Self-massage and swishing with coconut oil
- Tongue scraping
- Rinsing the eyes with cool water, and maybe rose water
- Yoga: learn some cooling sequences and breathing techniques from a skilled yoga teacher

- Meditation, like empty bowl or loving kindness meditations
- Take extra time for rest and relaxation … make time to PLAY!

3. Cultivate a lifestyle that balances the qualities of summer.

Explore the following guidelines to support balance and health during the summer:

- Stay cool.
- Wear a hat when outdoors.
- Use sunglasses when there is glare or bright sun.
- Keep the skin covered and wear loose silk and cotton clothes.
- Go for a swim.
- Sit in the shade and take in the sights and sounds of nature.
- Apply coconut oil to the feet and scalp at bedtime.
- Make time for fun, play, and good company.

4. Know what to reduce in the summer.

Avoid the following in the summertime:

- Hot, spicy, oily foods
- Excessive sour, salty, and pungent foods
- Large meals
- Skipping meals or fasting
- Drinking iced or hot drinks

- Smoking
- Exposure to the sun in the middle of the day
- Alcohol consumption (alcohol, generally speaking, is heating)
- Arguments, serious discussions, and the company of critical people

Recommendations for Fall

1. Choose a fall season balancing diet.

Here is how we approach our diet in the fall season:

- Favour warm, moist, heavy foods. It is the season of soups, stews, and casseroles. Which is great, because we tend to naturally crave these at this time of year ('cause our body knows!).
- Eat more sweet, salty, and sour foods. Please remember that sweet doesn't mean dessert. Think more along the lines of baked spiced fruit, like apple crisp.
- Eat lunch as the biggest meal to keep your digestion strong and your body warm.
- Keep hydrated with warm liquids, including warm water and tea.
- Great teas for the fall season include ginger, turmeric, chai, and tulsi.
- Reduce stimulants, like coffee and alcohol.

Specific fall balancing foods include:

- Meats: beef, chicken, duck, eggs, fish, lamb, pork, turkey, venison

- Grains (heavy and moistening): oatmeal, rice, wheat, and yeast-free breads
- Legumes: split yellow mung beans (sometimes these are spelled "moong")
- Fruits: cooked (baked is nice)—apples, bananas, berries, cranberries, dates, figs, grapefruit, lemons, limes, mangos, orange, papaya, peaches, and tangerine
- Veggies: carrots, sweet potatoes, beets, squash, pumpkins, garlic, tomatoes
- Favour warm milk drinks and *ghee* and increase healthy oils

2. Focus on important self-care routines for fall.

Here are the most useful routines for balancing your system in the fall season:

- Regular rhythm of waking, exercise (a.m.), mealtimes, and sleep
- Get plenty of sleep and rest—this is not the season to overwork or overdo
- Self-oil massage with warm sesame or sweet almond oil
- Oil your ears
- Nasal cleansing using a *neti* pot with salt water
- Oil your nostrils
- Yoga: learn a grounding, warming practice and how to work with the alternate nostril breath from a qualified yoga teacher
- Meditation, like Yoga Nidra or *mantra* repetition

3. Cultivate a lifestyle that balances the qualities of fall.

Explore the following guidelines to support balance and health during the fall:

- Wake up before the sun while the environment is still calm.
- Nurture your body (e.g., daily oil massage).
- Stay warm.
- Establish routines.
- Let go of hard workouts.
- Engage in more creative work.
- Enjoy calming activities.
- Reduce multitasking.
- Rest, nap, and enjoy quiet time.
- Cultivate gratitude by giving thanks.
- Create a safe environment for yourself.

4. Know what to reduce in the fall.

Here are the "don'ts" for fall:

- Dry brushing
- Raw, cold, dry, rough foods
- Cold or iced drinks ... cold or iced anything for that matter!
- Skipping meals or fasting
- Excessive snacking between meals
- Exposure to cold winds and drafts

- Excessive pungent, bitter, and astringent tastes
- Late nights
- Excessive sexual activity
- Switching from hot to cold and cold to hot

Recommendations for Winter

As previously discussed, winter in North America is interesting through the lens of the qualities. The cold quality continues to increase, accumulate, and aggravate, yet the accompanying qualities differ from winter to winter. When the winters are cold and dry, we continue to follow the regimen prescribed for fall. If the winter is cold and moist, then we follow the regimen prescribed for spring.

Putting the Daily Routine Together

It seems like a lot, doesn't it? And it is. There are a lot of options for each of us to take steps in the direction of our health. When I work with clients, I suggest they pick one thing and try it for a month and pay attention to what changes as a result of the recommendation. If you feel stronger, healthier, and more balanced—keep doing it. If not, maybe let it go. Then choose another recommendation and "wash, rinse, repeat." It's been my experience that very few people can make all the changes at once and keep doing it. Usually, too much change all at the same time leads to overwhelm and burnout. From here, we go back to our old way of doing things because it's what we can handle. So try one thing at a time and see if that works.

Folks start trying recommendations in one of two ways:

1. Something simple, easy, and totally doable for instant success. If you can find one of these, pick it!

2. Something necessary. If you picked up this book because you're having a hard time sleeping, then go back to the section on sleep and start working through those recommendations.

Both of these approaches are valid. You do you.

I've put together a cheat sheet for the daily routine to help you figure out what you're already doing, when you're doing it, and where it might make the most sense to start. You can download a fresh .pdf copy from my website (for free) so that you can print as many copies as you need to track your progress, if that works for you. Here's a sample of the Daily Routine Weekly Checklist on the following pages:

Morning Routine	MON	TUES	WED	THUR	FRI	SAT	SUN
1 Wake up (time)							
2 • Bathroom:							
• Elimination (pee and poop)							
• Scrape Tongue							
• Brush Teeth							
• Gargle, rinse, or swish							
• Rinse Eyes							
3 Cup of warm water (with lemon?)							
4 Movement (walking, yoga, etc.)							
5 Contemplation (meditation, journaling, etc.)							
6 Bathroom:							
• Dry Brush							
• Oil skin (massage)							
• Nose: neti & oil							
• Ears: oil							
• Shower/Bath							
7 Breakfast							
8 Life (work, play, etc.)							

Lunch Routine	MON	TUES	WED	THUR	FRI	SAT	SUN
1 Lunch as the largest meal							
2 Rest after eating							
3 100 steps							
4 Life (work, play, etc.)							

Dinner Routine		MON	TUES	WED	THUR	FRI	SAT	SUN
1	Lighter dinner							
2	Rest after eating							
3	100 steps							
4	Finish dinner two hours before bed							

Pre-Bed Routine		MON	TUES	WED	THUR	FRI	SAT	SUN
1	Get things ready for tomorrow							
2	Unplug: turn off the tech/screens							
3	Bathroom:							
	• Brush teeth & floss							
	• Gargle, rinse, or swish							
	• Oil							
	• Elimination							
4	Warm spiced milk or herbal tea							
5	Foot massage with warm oil							
6	Gentle stretching or meditation							
7	Bedtime							

CHAPTER 12

CONCLUSION TO PILLAR 3

The main idea behind this third pillar of energy management is figuring out how much energy you have and living within that amount of energy. The Ayurvedic daily routine, this structure, is useful and supports you in maintaining the energy and *ojas* you have, as well as building them. The daily routine is what pulls the whole book together. It helps keep your *agni* strong so you can build healthy tissues and *ojas*. It creates the space to eliminate *ama* and natural wastes from the body-mind. It helps with restorative sleep and creates awareness around how to manage your energy. It's the whole shebang!

It takes time, as well as trial and error, to figure out the daily routine that works for you, yet know that it is well worth the effort invested. If you get stuck sorting out the details for yourself, this is where working with someone one-on-one can be immensely useful. I have been working on my daily routine for over a decade now, and in that process, I have learned a lot of tips and tricks that have worked for my clients and me. I have also been through different iterations based on my changing needs at different times in my life.

Much like life and health are process-oriented, so is the daily routine.

One last thing about the daily routine: know that the attitude you bring to your self-care routine matters. If you treat it like one more "to do," then you will get some benefit from it; however, if you treat it as a ritual of health and self-love, you will get so much more benefit from it. Your intentions have impact. The choice of which intention you want to put behind your actions is yours to make.

Now that you have read this section, consider the following:

1. What are you already doing to manage your energy? Remember to keep this!

2. What is one thing you could do to support your energy?

3. Which aspects of the daily routine are already in place for you?

4. What could you explore to create more stability and support through your daily routine?

Epilogue

What a journey this Ayurvedic map has taken us on! Ayurveda has so much to teach us about maintaining our health. And yet it all comes down to choice. What step are you going to take in the direction of your health today?

Many different teachings, from physics[53] to philosophy,[54] understand that for each action we take an effect is produced. Another way to say this is that for each choice we make, there is a consequence. The word *consequence* often has ominous connotations; however, it actually depends on the consequence. Making choices that move us, one choice at a time, one step at a time, in the direction of our health leads us to wonderful consequences! Not all diseases are curable, yet a lot of them are preventable, if we choose health.

Our health is important not only to ourselves, but to the whole planet. Ayurveda teaches us that we are not separate from nature but an integrated part of the whole system. Where each of us finds balance, peace, and harmony, the whole system gets to experience it. Where humans choose health, the whole planet is healthier.

Ayurveda has given us a clear map with three pillars of health:

- Pillar 1—Nourishment: supporting our digestive fire to optimize nutritional intake so we can build strong healthy tissues, reducing metabolic waste production

---

53 Law of "action reaction."

54 Law of Karma.

to lower the risk of disease, and eliminating wastes from our system. It's not only what you eat, but how you eat it and if you digest it.

- Pillar 2—Sleep: the importance of restorative sleep for digestion (in body and mind), clearing out of toxins, rebuilding healthy tissues, and refilling the well of energy.

- Pillar 3—Energy management: understanding how much energy you have, knowing what uses it up, and implementing a daily routine to maintain and build your energy and resilience. Know your limit, play within it. Also, health is created by daily choices, not by chance. The best way to live healthy is to create a healthy daily routine where your health needs (diet, lifestyle, sleep) are met.

One of the most beautiful things about the three pillars is that they do not stand alone; they are interconnected, and they support each other. Nourishment allows you to sleep well and have energy to manage. Sleep supports digestion/ nourishment and energy management. Energy management supports digestion and sleep. They are the three legs of the stool of health (poop pun intended!). If any one of the pillars is not strong, then the stool falls over. The flip side to this is that you can start strengthening any of the pillars, and it supports the strengthening of all the pillars!

Even though the mind likes to make health complicated, it can be simple and straightforward. Every step you take in the direction of your health is a step in the direction of your health. The choice is always yours. Which step in the direction of your health will you take today?

Yours in health and with love (to build your *ojas*),

m xo

APPENDIX:

RECOMMENDATIONS LIST

I thought some of you might find it helpful to review the recommendations in a different way. In the book, I present the content and make recommendations, some of which are repeated along the way. In the table below, you'll find a list of all the recommendations without repetition as well as a column that shows you what the recommendation does. You will notice in this format that one recommendation can work on many things all at once, and this might influence your choices.

I hope this is useful to you. Enjoy!

#	Recommendation	What does this recommendation do?
1	Tongue scraping	Sense organ care—Mouth Removes *ama* Energy management
2	Teeth brushing	Sense organ care—Mouth Removes *ama* Energy management
3	Oil holding	Sense organ care—Mouth Removes *ama* Energy management
4	Swishing	Sense organ care—Mouth Removes *ama* Energy management
5	Gargling	Sense organ care—Mouth Removes *ama* or Nourish/build/strengthen tissues Energy management

#	Recommendation	What does this recommendation do?
6	Nasal rinsing using a *neti* pot and salt water	Sense organ care—Nose Removes *ama* Energy management
7	Oil your nostrils	Sense organ care—Nose Nourish/build/strengthen tissues Energy management
8	Eye rinse	Sense organ care—Eyes Removes *ama* Energy management
9	Rose water	Sense organ care—Eyes
10	Triphala infusion	Sense organ care—Eyes Removes *ama*
11	*Ghee*	Sense organ care—Eyes
12	Oil your ears	Sense organ care—Ears Nourish/build/strengthen tissues Energy management
13	Dry brushing	Sense organ care—skin Circulation—lymph/plasma Nourish/build/strengthen tissues Energy management
14	Self-oil massage	Sense organ care—skin Circulation Nourish/build/strengthen tissues Calms nerves *Ojas*-building Sweating Energy management
15	Daily shower/bath	Sense organ care—skin Removes *ama* Energy management
16	Daily sweating	Sense organ care—skin Removes *ama* Sweating

#	Recommendation	What does this recommendation do?
17	Meditation, including Yoga Nidra	Mind care Removes *ama* Nourishes/builds/strengthens Calms nerves Sleep hygiene Energy management
18	Time in nature	Mind care Removes *ama* Nourishes/builds/strengthens Calms nerves Supports digestion *Ojas*-building
19	Positive affirmations or *mantra*	Mind care Removes *ama* Nourishes/builds/strengthens Calms nerves Supports digestion
20	Favour warm cooked foods and avoid ice	*Agni*-boosting *Ama*-busting *Ojas*-building
21	Lunch as the largest meal of the day	*Agni*-boosting *Ama*-busting *Ojas*-building Energy management
22	Include all six tastes in your diet	*Agni*-boosting *Ama*-busting
23	When eating, focus on your food	*Agni*-boosting *Ama*-busting *Ojas*-building
24	When hunger arises, eat	*Agni*-boosting *Ama*-busting *Ojas*-building

#	Recommendation	What does this recommendation do?
25	Use ginger to stoke your *agni*: • Ginger pizzas • Ginger tea • Ginger juice mix	*Agni*-boosting *Ama*-busting
26	Eat until you are no longer hungry	*Agni*-boosting *Ama*-busting
27	Rest briefly after eating	*Agni*-boosting *Ama*-busting *Ojas*-building Energy management
28	Movement: daily exercise and activity	*Agni*-boosting *Ama*-busting Circulation—lymph/plasma Muscle-building Bowel movements Sweating Energy management
29	Daily routine—consistent: • Wake time • Morning routine • Meal times • Pre-bed routine • Bedtime	*Agni*-boosting *Ama*-busting Calms nerves Reproductive-building *Ojas*-building Sleep hygiene Energy management
30	Stay hydrated: drink enough water • Boiled water • Homemade healthy hydration drink	*Agni*-boosting *Ama*-busting Plasma/lymph building Bowel movements Urination Sweating

#	Recommendation	What does this recommendation do?
31	Choose a supportive eating environment	*Agni*-boosting *Ama*-busting Calms nerves *Ojas*-building Mind care
32	Sit to eat	*Agni*-boosting *Ama*-busting Calms nerves
33	Eat in a calm and peaceful environment	*Agni*-boosting *Ama*-busting Calms nerves *Ojas*-building Mind care
34	Eat in a clean space (*sattvic*)	*Agni*-boosting *Ama*-busting Calms nerves *Ojas*-building Mind care
35	Have something nice to look at	*Agni*-boosting *Ama*-busting Calms nerves *Ojas*-building Mind care
36	Be present and mindful (mindful eating)	*Agni*-boosting *Ama*-busting Calms nerves *Ojas*-building Mind care
37	Take a break while eating	*Agni*-boosting *Ama*-busting Calms nerves *Ojas*-building Mind care

#	Recommendation	What does this recommendation do?
38	Have an herbal tea after eating	*Agni*-boosting *Ama*-busting Calms nerves *Ojas*-building
39	Strengthen your *agni*	*Agni*-boosting *Ama*-busting **Builds ALL tissues including *OJAS*! Sweating
40	Reduce anything undigestible	*Ama*-busting
41	Avoid overconsumption	*Agni*-boosting *Ama*-busting
42	Choose simple, light, easy-to-digest foods	*Agni*-boosting *Ama*-busting
43	Reduce fast food, processed food, foods with additives (if you can't pronounce it, don't eat it) leftovers, canned and frozen foods	*Ama*-busting
44	Use basic food combining	*Agni*-boosting *Ama*-busting
45	Drink a cup of warm (or room temperature) water first thing	*Agni*-boosting *Ama*-busting Energy management
46	Drink CCF tea	*Agni*-boosting *Ama*-busting
47	Alternate nostril breathing	*Ama*-busting Calms nerves *Ojas*-building
48	Eat white foods	Plasma/lymph-building

#	Recommendation	What does this recommendation do?
49	Eat red and green foods	Blood-building
50	Drink nettle tea	Blood-building
51	Mindful three-part breathing	Blood-building Circulating—lymph/plasma
52	Eat grains, nuts, meat, and legumes	Muscle-building
53	Relax your muscles	Muscle-balancing Calms nerves
54	Eat healthy fats	Adipose-building Nerve/marrow-building
55	Bone broth	Bone-building
56	Weight-bearing exercise	Bone-building
57	Reduce your consumption of refined white sugar	Bone-building
58	Dark chocolate	Nerve-building
59	Calm your nerves	Calms nerves Bowel movements Urination
60	Eat sweet nourishing foods	Reproductive building
61	*Ojas*-building foods	*Ojas*-building
62	Retreat	*Ojas*-building
63	Media fasting—minimize screen time	Mind care *Ojas*-building Sleep hygiene
64	Reduce stress	*Ojas*-building Calms nerves Energy management

#	Recommendation	What does this recommendation do?
65	Yoga	*Ojas*-building Energy management
66	Work with your emotions	*Ojas*-building Heart-mind balancing
67	Aromatherapy	Calms nerves *Ojas*-building
68	Cultivate joy	*Ojas*-building Heart-mind balancing
69	Seek out beauty	*Ojas*-building
70	Animals (cuddles)	*Ojas*-building
71	Good work	*Ojas*-building Heart-mind balancing
72	Good company	*Ojas*-building Heart-mind balancing
73	Sweet words	*Ojas*-building Heart-mind balancing
74	Hugs	*Ojas*-building Heart-mind balancing
75	Laughter	*Ojas*-building Heart-mind balancing
76	Love (self, others, everyone)	*Ojas*-building Heart-mind balancing
77	Eliminate *ojas*-depleting factors	*Ojas*-preserving
78	When the urge to poop arises, go poop!	Bowel movement
79	When the urge to urinate arises, go pee!	Urination
80	Post-urination bladder squeeze	Urination
81	Consistent bedtime	Sleep hygiene

#	Recommendation	What does this recommendation do?
82	Keep your bedroom dark for sleep	Sleep hygiene
83	Bedroom for sleep and sex only	Sleep hygiene
84	Finish dinner two hours before bed	Sleep hygiene
85	Avoid stimulants before bed	Sleep hygiene
86	Herbal tea or warm spiced milk	Sleep hygiene *Agni*-boosting
87	Self foot massage w/ warm oil	Sleep hygiene
88	Wake before the sun rises	Energy management
89	Morning elimination of feces and urine	Energy management
90	Eat breakfast	Energy management
91	Take 100 steps after a meal	*Agni*-boosting Energy management
92	Eat a lighter dinner	*Agni*-boosting *Ama*-busting Energy management
93	Get things ready for tomorrow	Energy management Sleep hygiene
94	Spring diet, foods, self-care regimens, lifestyle	Everything!
95	Summer diet, foods, self-care regimens, lifestyle	Everything!
96	Fall diet, foods, self-care regimens, lifestyle	Everything!

Further Reading

Ayurveda References

Brown, Christina. *The Ayurvedic Year*. North Adams: Storey Books, 2002.

Charaka + Sharma, Dr. Ram Karan and Dash, Vaidya Bhagwan (translations & commentaries by). *Charaka Samhita*. Varanasi India: Chowkhamba Press, 2014.

Douillard, Dr. John. *The 3-Season Diet*. New York: Three Rivers Press, 2000.

Frawley, Dr. David. *Ayurveda and the Mind: The Healing of Consciousness*. Twin Lakes: Lotus Press, 1997.

Kripalu School of Ayurveda. *Kripalu School of Ayurveda— Foundations of Ayurveda Student Manual*, 2012.

Lad, Dr. Vasant. *Ayurveda—The Science of Self-Healing*. Twin Lakes: Lotus Press, 2009.

Lad, Dr. Vasant. *Textbook of Ayurveda Fundamental Principles Volume 1*. Albuquerque: The Ayurvedic Press, 2002.

O'Donnell, Kate. *The Everyday Ayurveda Cookbook*. Boston: Shambhala, 2015.

Svoboda, Dr. Robert. *Prakriti*. Twin Lakes: Lotus Press, 1998.

"The Elements and their Attributes." *Vibrational Ayurveda* (website). June 19, 2018. http://vibrationalAyurveda.com /new-page-1/.

Vagbhata + Murthy, K R Srikantha. *Ashtanga Samgraha*. Varanasi India: Chowkhamba Orientalia, 2013.

Vagbhata + Murthy, K R Srikantha. *Ashtanga Hrdayam*. Varanasi India: Chowkhamba Press, 2013.

Welch, Dr. Claudia. *Balance Your Hormones, Balance Your Life*. Cambridge: Da Capo Press, 2011.

Dharma/Life Purpose References

Chokoisky, Simon. *The Five Dharma Types*. Vermont: Destiny Books, 2012.

Cope, Stephen. *The Great Work of Your Life*. New York: Bantam Books, 2012.

Establishing New Habits Reference

Rubin, Gretchen. *Better Than Before.* Canada: Anchor Canada, 2015.

Bibliography

"Big." Google. Accessed March 2018. https://www.google.ca/se arch?q=Dictionary.

Charaka + Sharma, Dr. Ram Karan and Dash, Vaidya Bhagwan (translations & commentaries by). *Charaka Samhita.* Varanasi India: Chowkhamba Press, 2014.

Chödrön, Pema. *Getting Unstuck.* Sounds True, 2005.

"Clear." Google. Accessed March 2018. https://www.google.ca /search?q=Dictionary.

"Cloudy." Google. Accessed March 2018. https://www.google .ca/search?q=Dictionary.

"Cold." Google. Accessed March 2018. https://www.google.ca /search?q=Dictionary.

"Dense." Google. Accessed March 2018. https://www.google.ca /search?q=Dictionary.

"Dilution." Google. Accessed March 2018. https://www.google .ca/search?q=Dictionary.

"Dry." Google. Accessed March 2018. https://www.google.ca/se arch?q=Dictionary.

"Dull." Google. Accessed March 2018, https://www.google.ca /search?q=Dictionary.

"Gross." Google. Accessed March 2018. https://www.google.ca /search?q=Dictionary.

"Hard." Google. Accessed March 2018. https://www.google.ca /search?q=Dictionary.

"Heavy." Google. Accessed March 2018. https://www.google.ca /search?q=Dictionary.

"Hot." Google. Accessed March 2018. https://www.google.ca/se arch?q=Dictionary.

Lad, Dr. Vasant. *Textbook of Ayurveda Fundamental Principles Volume 1.* Albuquerque: The Ayurvedic Press, 2002.

"Light." Google. Accessed March 2018, https://www.google.ca /search?q=Dictionary.

"Liquid." Google. Accessed March 2018. https://www.google.ca /search?q=Dictionary.

"Mobile." Google. Accessed March 2018. https://www.google.ca /search?q=Dictionary.

"Obvious." Google. Accessed March 2018. https://www.google .ca/search?q=Dictionary.

"Oily." Google. Accessed March 2018. https://www.google.ca/se arch?q=Dictionary.

"Penetrating." Google. Accessed March 2018. https://www.go ogle.ca/search?q=Dictionary.

"Rough." Google. Accessed March 2018. https://www.google.ca /search?q=Dictionary.

"Sharp." Google. Accessed March 2018. https://www.google.ca /search?q=Dictionary.

"Slimy." Google. Accessed March 2018. https://www.google.ca /search?q=Dictionary.

"Slow." Google. Accessed March 2018, https://www.google.ca /search?q=Dictionary.

"Smooth." Google. Accessed March 2018. https://www.google .ca/search?q=Dictionary.

"Soft." Google. Accessed March 2018. https://www.google.ca
/search?q=Dictionary.

"Spread." Google. Accessed January 2019. https://www.google
.ca/search?q=Dictionary.

"Stable." Google. Accessed March 2018. https://www.google.ca
/search?q=Dictionary.

"Sticky." Google. Accessed March 2018. https://www.google.ca
/search?q=Dictionary.

"Subtle." Google. Accessed March 2018. https://www.google.ca
/search?q=Dictionary.

"The densest objects in the universe." ESA. Updated Oct. 15,
2002. http://www.esa.int/Our_Activities/Space_Science/In
tegral/The_densest_objects_in_the_Universe.

Vagbhata + Murthy, K R Srikantha. *Ashtanga Samgraha*.
Varanasi India: Chowkhamba Orientalia, 2013.

Vagbhata + Murthy, K R Srikantha. *Ashtanga Hrdayam*. Varanasi
India: Chowkhamba Press, 2013.

Gratitude

To Gummo, this is your book. You're the one who said, "When you're writing the book on Ayurvedic Yoga and there are all these things you want to say, but they don't fit in the first book. Those things will become a second book, and that's the one I want to read." You totally called it. I hope you enjoyed it as much as I did. 🖤

To V, who answers a million questions, did the second proof-read despite the busiest life and schedule ever, and provides tons of guidance and support. Thank you for the deep review of the content, the great suggestions, and everything you do for me all the time. I love you, my sister from another mister. 🖤

To my round-one proofreaders: Gummo, Sarah K, Dr. Sonya, and Maggie. Your feedback greatly improved this book in so many ways—thank you so very much! I am grateful to each of you for making the most vulnerable part of this process safe and loving for me. I am grateful to have strong, brilliant friends and family surrounding me. 🖤

To my Ayurveda teachers, Dr. Anusha, Larissa, Dr. Rosy, Dr. Claudia, Dr. Margrit, Dr. Scott, Dr. Satyanarayan Dasa, Dr. John, Dr. Jyothi, Dr. Lad, Dr. Joshi, Dr. Svoboda, and Dr. Frawley. Thank you for sharing your Ayurvedic wisdom. I hope I honoured what you shared and taught. That was my intention. In particular, I want to thank Dr. Anusha, who spent time with me to clarify many small details about many different aspects of Ayurveda and its practice, as well as supported me in finding references from the classical texts to include. I am so grateful, Anushaji. 🖤

To my teacher Siobhan. Thank you for years of ongoing support. For helping me to be courageous and inviting me to step into authorship (and everything that goes with it). Thank you for inviting me to understand more deeply, for sharing your wisdom, and for reminding me to share the teachings with integrity from my heart. ♥

To my clients and students, who want to learn Ayurveda, and who inspire me to want to teach it better. Thank you for showing up. Without you, there's nothing. ♥

To the team at Janati Yoga School: Thank you for your love and support. I love that we are Janatians. ♥

To the team at Archangel Ink for helping this book be the best and most useful it can be. Kristie Lynn, Paige, Vanessa, Tyler, Rob, and everyone else: I am grateful for your care, expertise, and patience. ♥

To my parents, who have supported everything I've ever done for my whole life. Thank you for loving me no matter what. I noticed. It matters. I love you back, no matter what. ♥

To my husband, Glenn, who is the love of my life, my best friend, and my home. Thank you for booking me a writing retreat so I could finish this book. Thank you for creating the space in our life for this bumpy trek that definitely did not follow "the plan." I love you, my babeh. ♥

To the Vedas and sages, thank you for these teachings. They have changed my life and made me a better person. I am eternally grateful for your existence and to live in a time when I have access to these rich lessons. *OM.*

Resources

Obviously, I'm into Ayurveda. As a result, my website (http://www.janatiyoga.com) has a lot of different opportunities for you to explore further:

- Free Introduction to Ayurveda Online course
- Fall 9-day Digestive Reset Program Online (fall only)
- Spring 1-month Digestive Reset Program Online (spring only)
- Postpartum Ayurvedic Self-Care for Mama Online
- Ayurvedic Yoga video classes (*doshic, yin, agni, ojas, sattva*)
- Yoga Nidra meditation (audio files)

As a thank you for reading the book this far, please enjoy the following coupon code for 15% off any audio or video classes from the website: **A3POHbook15**

If you're looking to find someone near you to help you on your Ayurveda journey, check the following websites as a starting place:

- National Ayurvedic Medical Association (US & Canada): https://www.ayurvedanama.org/
- Ayurveda Association of Canada (Canada): https://ayurvedaassociation.ca/

I don't know any organizations off my own continent at this time. If you can't find anyone near you, I offer consultations online via Zoom and would be happy to work with you. You can send me an email at mona@monawarner.com.

I love to teach, and my husband loves to travel. If you want me to come to you to offer a workshop, retreat, or lecture, please reach out!

A Humble Request

If you enjoyed this book and learned something from it, it would be amazing if you could share your thoughts on Amazon or email me your feedback. Your honest and sincere review will help others who would benefit from this information to find it more easily. My publishers tell me that it helps more than I can understand.

Thank you for considering.

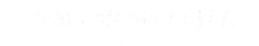

About the Author

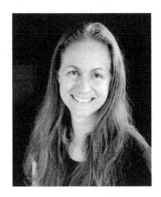

Mona Warner is a warm and joyful educator. Her depth of knowledge, passion, and dedication to the practices of yoga and Ayurveda are evident. Mona leads by example, encouraging students to be and honour themselves, their practice, and others.

Mona works at the Janati Yoga School in Kingston, Ontario, Canada, where she lives with her wonderful husband, enthusiastic dog, and ninja kitten. She has been practicing yoga since 2001, teaching yoga since 2004, and teaching Ayurveda since 2013. She is a Registered Yoga Teacher Trainer with the Yoga Alliance (ERYT500), a National Ayurvedic Medical Association recognized Ayurvedic Yoga Therapist (AYT-NAMA), and a Certified Ayurvedic Practitioner (CAP-NAMA). She is also the author of Ayurvedic Yoga.

When she's not practicing, teaching, or talking about Vedic Sciences, you might find her eating chocolate, reading a book on a beach, climbing a mountain in Ireland, kayaking up to glaciers in Alaska, or zip lining in Costa Rica. But mostly, you'll find her eating chocolate.

Made in the
USA
Middletown, DE